'I am delighted to see this book actually based on what health and social care professionals want to know about dementia care. The chapters use complex and challenging case studies or related examples, with expert navigation and advice from an experienced Admiral Nurse to add context, guidance and understanding. As a result, the Admiral Nurses and their colleagues have produced a really useful practical text which I hope will get the wide readership it truly deserves.'

– Professor Martin Orrell, Director of the Institute of
Mental Health, University of Nottingham

'Drawing directly from the specialist skills, values and practice knowledge of Admiral Nurses, this accessible book is a treasure trove of (in) valuable information for generalist practitioners working with, and alongside, people affected by dementia in any environment of care. It is essential reading.'

– John Keady, Professor of Mental Health Nursing and
Older People, The University of Manchester

'Highly practical, exceedingly well-informed, clearly relevant to day-to-day practice, this book provides a useful and stimulating resource for those, in many different circumstances, who work with people living with dementia. This should be no surprise, given the standing of the Admiral Nurses who have contributed their wisdom to these pages.'

– Julian C. Hughes, Honorary Professor,
Bristol Medical School, University of Bristol

'A great book based on the experiences of health and care professionals that tackles all the big questions about how to respond and support people living with dementia when it might not be your area of expertise. Everyone working in health and social care would learn something new from reading this book.'

– Claire Goodman, Professor of Health Care Research,
University of Hertfordshire

What You *Really* Want to Know About Working with Dementia

Real Issues and Expert Advice

KAREN HARRISON DENING,
HILDA HAYO AND AMY PEPPER

Foreword by Jan Oyebode

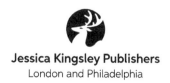

Jessica Kingsley Publishers
London and Philadelphia

First published in Great Britain in 2025 by Jessica Kingsley Publishers
An imprint of John Murray Press

1

Copyright unless otherwise stated © Karen Harrison
Dening, Hilda Hayo and Amy Pepper 2025

Foreword copyright © Jan Oyebode 2025

Copyright of contributions in the following chapters: Chapter 1: Amy Pepper
and Laura Maio 2025; Chapter 2: Liz Watret and Beth Goss-Hill 2025; Chapter 3:
Joanne Bush and Lucy Chamberlain 2025; Chapter 4: Sarra Blackman and Emma
Wolverson 2025; Chapter 5: Amy Kerti 2025; Chapter 6: Sarra Blackman and Nikki
Rowe 2025; Chapter 7: Deiondre Jackson and Zena Aldridge 2025; Chapter 8: Jenny
Butler and Caroline Scates 2025; Chapter 9: Melissa O'Reilly, Alexa Durham and
Chris O'Connor 2025; Chapter 10: Ella Balmer and Kerry Lyons 2025; Chapter 11:
Serenity Underhill and Jane Pritchard 2025; Chapter 12: Julie Bentham and Victoria
Davies 2025; Chapter 13: Alison Holden and Joanne Freeman 2025; Chapter 14:
Anthony MacKay and Kerry Lyons 2025; Chapter 15: Sophie Wellman and Kerry
Lyons 2025; Chapter 16: Shiny Varghese and Dio Giotas 2025; Chapter 17: Elizabeth
Jenkins and Sharron Tolman 2025; Chapter 18: Alison Stewart and Laura Birch 2025

A CIP catalogue record for this title is available from the
British Library and the Library of Congress

ISBN 978 1 83997 636 0
eISBN 978 1 83997 637 7

Printed and bound in Great Britain by CPI Group (UK)

Jessica Kingsley Publishers' policy is to use papers that are natural,
renewable and recyclable products and made from wood grown in
sustainable forests. The logging and manufacturing processes are expected
to conform to the environmental regulations of the country of origin.

Jessica Kingsley Publishers
Carmelite House
50 Victoria Embankment
London EC4Y 0DZ

www.jkp.com

John Murray Press
Part of Hodder & Stoughton Ltd
An Hachette Company

The authorised representative in the EEA is Hachette Ireland, 8 Castlecourt
Centre, Castleknock Road, Castleknock, Dublin 15, D15 YF6A, Ireland

Contents

Meet the editors

DR KAREN HARRISON DENING

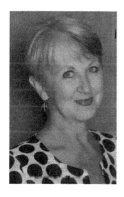

Karen has over 45 years' experience in nursing, most of those being in dementia care in a variety of settings and contexts. She is Head of Research and Publications at Dementia UK. She gained her PhD at UCL in advance care planning and end-of-life care in dementia. Through her role at Dementia UK, she is a collaborator, co-applicant and expert advisor to several national and international research studies. She served on the National Institute for Health and Care Excellence (NICE) dementia guideline committees. Her research interests include dementia care, case management, carer resilience, palliative and end-of-life care, and advance care planning.

DR HILDA HAYO

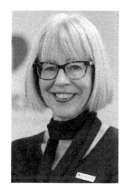

Hilda became Chief Admiral Nurse and CEO for Dementia UK in 2013. A dual registered nurse, over the last 36 years she has held senior positions in clinical services, hospital management and higher education. Hilda is particularly proud of setting up and leading a nurse-led Younger People with Dementia service in Northamptonshire and still provides specialist advice and support to families. Her doctorate focused on behavioural variant frontotemporal dementia and how this affects families. She has also written a book on *Young Onset Dementia* with two colleagues published in 2018.

AMY PEPPER

Amy qualified as a mental health nurse in 2008 and specialized in dementia care, working in a number of care settings. In 2014 she developed and led the Admiral Nursing Service in the London Borough of Sutton, carrying out an evaluation that led to an increase in funding and expansion of the team. Following this she worked on the Admiral Nurse Dementia Helpline with the Research and Publications Team within Dementia UK. She currently works as a Dementia Care Manager for HC-One where 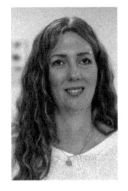 she provides clinical leadership to care and nursing homes She also continues to practice clinically as an Admiral Nurse on the Admiral Nurse Dementia Helpline.

Contributors to this book

HEALTH AND SOCIAL CARE PROFESSIONALS WORKING WITH PEOPLE WITH DEMENTIA AND FAMILY CARERS

- Zena Aldridge
- Ella Balmer
- Julie Bentham
- Sarra Blackman
- Joanne Bush
- Jenny Butler
- Alexa Durham
- Alison Holden
- Deiondre Jackson (pseudonym)
- Anthony MacKay
- Alison Stewart
- Melissa O'Reilly
- Serenity Underhill
- Shiny Varghese
- Liz Watret
- Sophie Wellman

DEMENTIA UK AND ADMIRAL NURSES

- Laura Birch
- Lucy Chamberlain
- Victoria Davies
- Joanne Freeman
- Dio Giotas
- Beth Goss-Hill
- Elizabeth Jenkins
- Amy Kerti
- Kerry Lyons
- Laura Maio
- Caroline Scates
- Chris O'Connor
- Dr Jane Pritchard
- Nikki Rowe
- Sharron Tolman
- Dr Emma Wolverson

Foreword

Jan Oyebode

The condition of dementia accompanies those with a diagnosis everywhere they go. Keith Oliver, a well-known ambassador for those living with the condition, has likened it to an unwelcome guest. If you live with dementia it is with you if a nurse comes from your GP practice to check up on your diabetes; it is with you if you have to go into hospital for cancer treatment. It is at home with you if a live-in carer comes to help you, and if you move into a care home, it moves in with you. This means it is vital for health and social care staff in all these settings to have the knowledge and skills to understand how dementia affects those they work with. They need to know how to find out about its impact on each unique individual and how to manage its impact as they seek to provide good care. In this book, Admiral Nurses bring invaluable clinical wisdom to bear on a whole range of situations and circumstances encountered by health and social care staff. It will be a treasure trove for all health and social care professionals who are not dementia specialists but who provide services to a population that includes some who have this unwelcome guest with them.

As a clinical psychologist working with older people, I was lucky enough to work alongside Admiral Nurses in mental health services for many years. In my experience, these specialist dementia care nurses bring exceptional commitment and deep expertise to bear in the support of people living with dementia and their families. In this context, I was delighted to be approached to write the foreword for this book, *What You Really Want to Know About Working with Dementia*. The book demonstrates that dementia care is 'everybody's business'. It shows that general health and social care professionals across a huge array of care settings want to know more about how to provide skilled support and care to meet the needs of people living with dementia and it clearly demonstrates that Admiral Nurses have hugely valuable clinical experience and a body of practice-based and evidence-based knowledge to pass on to colleagues across this wide range of settings.

What You Really *Want to Know About Working with Dementia* has an ingenious, engaging structure. The editors, Dr Karen Harrison Dening, Dr Hilda Hayo and Amy Pepper, hit on the idea of asking health and social care professionals what they wanted to know about dementia and dementia care. Professionals responded with examples of the challenges they face and the times they wished they had known more about what to do. The book picks up these issues chapter by chapter. Each starts with a case study or some examples from a health or care practitioner who is not a dementia specialist. These outline the dilemmas or situations they struggle with, and are followed by a commentary from an Admiral Nurse who draws out key aspects and offers knowledge and advice on possible strategies for managing the issues. This is therefore essentially a 'needs-led' text; its content being based entirely on what non-dementia specialist staff said they needed to know. It carries real-life validity and the cases will strike an immediate chord with others who work in these various settings.

The scenarios provide a spectrum of examples of situations staff find hard to manage, such as wondering whether 'therapeutic lies' should be preferred to absolute honesty; managing differences between family reactions to dementia; responding to needs of people in hospice care and general wards; and supporting older couples where both are frail. I was full of admiration for the generalist staff who put these cases forward. We see their compassion and their motivation to know more about dementia care as they reflect on their experiences. But it is the commentaries provided by the Admiral Nurses that are the heart of the book. The Admiral Nurses write from a person-centred, practice-informed perspective about how to approach these situations. They offer analysis, facts, thoughtful tips and pragmatic suggestions based not on academic learning but on real-world, in-depth experience. Admiral Nurses are not only found in dementia services but in many other settings too from palliative care to physical health hospitals, but they are still quite few and far between. This excellent text will bring their much-needed expertise to a wide audience of generalist health and social care staff.

Preface

Over the years in working with Dementia UK both as a Consultant Admiral Nurse based in the NHS and then in senior positions within the charity, I have been conscious of how much we support other colleagues in health and social care in their support of people with dementia and their family carers and supporters. I see it as an essential aspect of the role of Admiral Nursing and of the case management approach we offer. As well as each Admiral Nurse working in their own services and locality to support, educate and mentor a range of stakeholders, I have undertaken this role in a wider sense as I head Dementia UK's Research and Publications team. One aspect of my role is to support Admiral Nurses to write for publication and this can take many guises, such as blogs, book reviews, peer review journal articles and many other forms that illustrate their role and clinical activity. One of the most successful forms of publication has been Admiral Nurse case studies. The nurse will introduce the issue, for example diagnostic overshadowing, that often confounds generalist care when a person with dementia develops a co-morbid physical illness. This will then be discussed using an anonymized and illustrative case study from which it can be reflected upon based in evidence and best clinical practice.

During the last two years we have also been approached by several editors of nursing journals to write papers on aspects of dementia care which have then developed into a multiple article series. As the years pass, it can feel like we are repeating ourselves and writing on the same issues. Maybe this approach was not having the best impact? So, we decided to ask generalist clinicians in both health and social care what did *they* want to know. What were the issues for *them* as they support people with dementia and their family carers in clinical practice. Rather than the Admiral Nurse presenting their case study and examining the issues through their lens, we wanted to see the issues through the lens of generalist practitioners. As you read this book, you will see the diverse range of professionals that responded to our call for cases (see Chapter 1) and the sometimes-complex scenarios they face. We hope that by responding this way to your issues and concerns we can both inform and give confidence to the amazing work you do.

A note on the text: all of the names and some of the case details used in this book, in relation to case examples, have been fictionalized to anonymize the individuals referred to.

Dr Karen Harrison Dening

Admiral Nursing

Admiral Nurses are specialist dementia nurses who are continually supported and developed by Dementia UK and who provide life-changing support for families affected by all forms of dementia. The nurses work with the person with dementia, and their family, to identify their needs and a plan of care is then devised to meet these needs. Admiral Nurses provide specialist advice and support in order for the family to understand dementia, and to help them develop the knowledge, skills and confidence to manage their future with dementia. Management of complex issues, for example changes in roles and relationships, distress, decisions about accepting care and support, communication difficulties and changed behaviour or personality, are all areas that Admiral Nurses specialize in.

Admiral Nurses also provide specialist dementia education, leadership, development and support to other health and social care colleagues. In addition to being specialist dementia nurses, some Admiral Nurses also specialize in different areas of dementia including young onset dementia, Lewy body dementia, frailty, end-of-life care, diverse communities, learning disability, acute care, primary care and long-term care. This book highlights the work of some of our Admiral Nurses in a range of settings and provides an example of their specialist knowledge and skills in a range of situations.

So why are we called Admiral Nurses? The family of Joseph Levy CBE BEM – who founded the charity Dementia UK – named the nurses. Joseph had vascular dementia and was known affectionately as 'Admiral Joe' because of his love of sailing. His family wanted to make a difference for families living with the effects of dementia and set up the charity to support and develop specialist dementia nurses and decided to call us Admiral Nurses.

The number of Admiral Nurses across the UK is steadily increasing, and they work in a range of services including the community, GP practices, NHS hospitals, hospices and care homes. There are still areas of the UK that don't have access to a local Admiral Nurse service and for these families we have the Admiral Nurse Dementia Helpline (0800 888 6678 or email on helpline@dementiauk.org) open seven days per week and staffed entirely by specialist dementia nurses. In addition, we have Admiral Nurse Clinics where a virtual appointment can be booked with a specialist dementia nurse.

Dr Hilda Hayo, Chief Admiral Nurse and CEO Dementia UK

CHAPTER 1

Consultation is key

DEVELOPING THE BOOK

INTRODUCTION

In developing the content for this book, we sought the practice concerns and issues that health and social care professionals face when working with families with dementia. Understanding what most challenged the professionals' delivery of care enabled us to consider what information could be provided to enable them to both confidently and effectively care for people living with the impact of dementia on their caseloads. Whilst there are many specialist practitioners and services supporting families with dementia, a great deal of the care and support offered to families affected by dementia over the course of the condition will be provided by generalist practitioners. We know that, despite the drive to increase both awareness and knowledge of dementia (DH 2015), many still lack the training and the confidence needed to support the varied and often complex issues that a dementia diagnosis can bring (Parveen et al. 2021).

An important part of the role of an Admiral Nurse is to provide consultancy to other professionals, supporting them to increase their knowledge and skills in dementia care, and supporting the implementation of best practice in the areas in which they work (Harrison Dening, Aldridge et al. 2022). Admiral Nurses in the community, and on the Dementia Helpline and Clinics, provide what many textbooks about dementia do not. Admiral Nurses can answer the real-life questions that generalist practitioners struggle with as they support people and their families impacted by dementia on their caseloads. The aim of this book was to start from the perspective of the generalist practitioner and the areas of dementia care that *they* find problematic, and provide advice from Admiral Nurses around those issues.

UNDERSTANDING THE ISSUES AND CONCERNS

As stated, we wanted the contents of this book to be led by the real issues facing generalist practitioners, and with this in mind we carried out a national survey, exploring the areas that generalist practitioners find particularly challenging in their work with people, and their families, impacted by dementia. In addition to this we undertook an analysis of the Admiral Nurse Dementia Helpline data, where the caller was a health or social care professional, and used both sets of data to guide the book's content.

METHODS
Survey

We developed a survey tool that sought to understand the common issues generalist practitioners faced in managing their day-to-day caseload when the person had a co-morbid diagnosis of dementia. We provided a question with a drop-down list of prompts for areas of potential difficulty, such as compliance with treatments or medication, behaviours they found challenging, forgetfulness in their patients, as well as leaving the option to describe other issues that did not appear in the drop-down list. We also asked for anonymized demographic data including any dementia education or training they received, discipline, role and number of years in practice. We also asked if any of the respondents would be willing to share their issues or practice concerns through an anonymized, illustrative case study or story narrative that could form the basis of a book section. This was the format successfully used by the editors in a recent text – *What you really want to know about life with dementia* (Harrison Dening, Hayo et al. 2022).

The online survey tool was promoted through the CHAIN network (a network connecting health and social care practitioners), the Royal Colleges newsletters (nursing, OT, GP, etc.) and through editorials and news features in several nursing journals, such as *Journal of Clinical Nursing, Nursing Standard, British Journal of Neuroscience Nursing* and *Nursing Times*. The survey was open between February and May 2022.

Helpline data

We also looked at a sample of data from the Admiral Nurse Dementia Helpline between July 2021 and August 2022, looking specifically at contacts received from other professionals and the reasons for their calls.

RESULTS

Helpline data

There were a total of 1,103 professional contacts to the helpline during this period. Table 1.1 shows the types of professionals from whom calls were received during the time period.

Table 1.1: Breakdown of professional callers to the helpline by discipline

Professional	No. of contacts
Nurse	235
Social worker	166
Charity sector	145
Carer/HCA	135
Non-health professional	121
Care navigator/social prescriber	96
OT	55
Doctor	44
Hospice staff	28
Psychologist/therapist/counsellor	18
Police	16
Physiotherapist	10
Dietician	7
Paramedic	6
Researcher	5
Speech and language therapist	4
Audiologist	3
Dentist	3

cont.

Professional	No. of contacts
Pharmacist	2
Podiatrist	1
Other	3

We analysed the primary reason for the call (see Table 1.2). By far, the main request for support was for input from an Admiral Nurse to support their practice; second was how to access other supports for a family affected by dementia in their care; and third, to gain understanding about aspects of dementia care to support a person with dementia on their caseload.

Table 1.2: Top reasons for requests for support on the Admiral Nurse Dementia Helpline

Reason for call	Total
Wants an Admiral Nurse	512
Accessing support	385
Dementia understanding and support	108
General information about Admiral Nurses/Dementia UK	91

Survey data
We collected responses from 81 professionals; the majority (n=63, 78%) expressed difficulties whilst working with families affected by dementia.

Profile of respondents
Nurses represented the majority of the respondents (n=29, 46%), followed by allied health professionals (n=15, 23%); social care staff (n=9, 14%); and other professionals (n=8, 13%). Only two medical doctors (3%) participated in the survey. Other professionals included administrative or clerical staff; healthcare support workers; dementia link workers; and professional carers (see Figure 1.1).

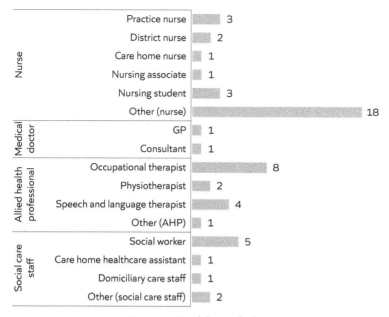

Figure 1.1: Breakdown of roles

Most respondents were based in an acute hospital setting (n=34, 54%). Respondents were also from community nursing and therapy (n=7, 11.1%), social care (9.5%) and mental health services (n=5, 7.9%).

There was a range of years worked in health and social care; from under one year to over 30 years. Almost 90% of respondents had received some form of training in dementia care, although the level varied widely from those who had accessed training provided by their employer to those who had undertaken undergraduate courses in dementia.

DIFFICULTIES ENCOUNTERED WHEN PROVIDING CARE TO PEOPLE WITH DEMENTIA AND/OR THEIR FAMILY CARERS

Many difficulties were reported in relation to providing care to people with dementia and their family carers, with the top two being *compliance with treatments/medication for other conditions* (83%) and a *family carer's health impacting on their caring role* (83%) (see Figure 1.2) (some respondents identified two or more difficulties).

Respondents could select more than one option

Person living with dementia's compliance with treatments/medication for other conditions	52,83%
Family carer's health impacting on their caring role	52,83%
Person living with dementia's behaviours you find challenging	50,79%
Managing families' expectations	50,79%
Family carer's lack of knowledge and/or understanding of dementia	45,71%
Lack of access to appropriate resources for a person and/or family affected by dementia	44,70%
Family carer's lack of acceptance of a diagnosis of dementia	41,65%
Managing nutrition and hydration in a person with dementia	41,65%
Person living with dementia's forgetfulness	39,62%
Difficulties in communicating with a person with dementia	39,62%
Managing risk of a person with dementia (e.g., driving, leaving their home at unsociable hours	38,60%

Figure 1.2: Top issues or difficulties when providing dementia care

THEMATIC ANALYSIS OF SURVEY RESPONSES

As well as the closed survey questions, respondents also had the opportunity to describe problems commonly encountered in their care of families affected by dementia. This provided us with qualitative data which was analysed thematically (Braun and Clarke 2022). The authors coded separately, then came together to compare and review, agreeing on revisions before identifying the themes which impact both the person with dementia and the staff. These were:

- gaps in services
- cognitive changes
- co-morbidities
- behaviours that challenge
- balancing risk/positive risk management
- working with family carers.

DISCUSSION
Gaps in services

Many spoke of a mismatch between the services available or funded and the support that was required by families they were supporting. This started from the point of seeking a diagnosis, with delays to diagnosis and misdiagnosis being highlighted. This mirrored survey responses (70%) that identified facilitating access to diagnostic services as a challenge in their practice.

> 'Often it is being able to get the diagnosis as [this] can be a lengthy process'.
> Nurse, acute hospital

There was limited, or sometimes an absence of, coordinated care and effective communication between health and social care systems, particularly in services to support transitions of care or in referrals to other services. Respondents felt the absence of such transitional care led to problems, such as delayed discharges from acute care, accessing social care and respite which often resulted in inappropriate admissions to care homes.

> 'Biggest problems tend to be in joined up communication between health and social services and patients/carers actually being able to get hold of staff to assist and facilitate signposting to correct agencies.'
> Nurse, community

> 'The biggest challenge is often coordination and accessing services.'
> Occupational Therapist, community

Sometimes these gaps were attributed to a lack of knowledge about dementia and dementia care, with decisions made by health and social care leaders often not being informed by the realities of the complexities of caring for people with dementia, leaving staff on the ground to 'manage the fallout', for example decisions around bed moves in acute hospital:

> 'People are placed in senior positions in the trust who do not have clinical experience leading to unsafe bed moves and beds being set up in unsafe environments for patients with dementia. Certain wards are forced to take large numbers of patients with dementia and extended needs without having any extra staffing provided to support this

meaning it is unsafe for patients with dementia. Ward staff are over stretched as it is.'
Nurse, acute care

Inadequate staffing levels, as alluded to in the quote above, also presented a significant challenge for many, with a knock-on impact on the ability to provide what was perceived to be meaningful occupation for people with dementia in some care settings.

Moving a person with dementia from one service or care setting to another was difficult at times. Cross service referrals were often not straightforward with professionals encountering several barriers, such as knowing the decision-making hierarchy of another service and their differing priorities sometimes being difficult to understand or navigate.

Respondents also reflected that the pandemic had exacerbated an already stretched system.

Cognitive changes

A difficulty experienced by generalist practitioners was the impact of cognitive changes on the person with dementia's ability to engage with appointments, treatment plans and advice given.

'Difficult...when person...keeps forgetting their appointments.'
Nurse, community

Almost 85% of respondents identified compliance with medication and treatments as being an area that presented management problems of other conditions co-morbid to their dementia, and this was reflected in the qualitative data, with 'medication administration' (Nurse, community) and 'overdose of medication' (Nurse, acute hospital) being particular problems.

Communication with the person with dementia was felt to be challenging at times:

'When end of life is approaching it can be challenging to communicate this to the patient due to their reduced capacity.'
Nurse, hospice

There were also difficulties encountered in how to manage a situation where the person with dementia lacked insight into their needs.

'...lack of compliance with recommendations due to either lack of understanding initially or being unable to recall advice...anything from use of equipment, taking meds, doing exercises, accepting carers...'.
Occupational Therapist, community

'Patients with dementia not understanding or remembering why they are in hospital, and this can make them panic'.
Nurse, acute hospital

Co-morbidities
Respondents related to the difficulties in managing complexity in the person with dementia when there was multi-morbidity, particularly in distinguishing between symptoms that were due to the dementia and those due to their other physical conditions.

'It's [dementia] such an intense condition which involves and affects different other conditions...it's very hard to tear them [each condition] apart or understand the process of dealing with one to help the other'.
Nurse, acute hospital

Behaviours that challenge
Although the preferred term is 'distressed behaviours', the theme title of 'behaviours that challenge' reflected the wording used by the respondents. Underpinning this theme were difficulties associated with a lack of knowledge and understanding about how to manage such behaviours, and in understanding their root causes:

'Often, if a service user displays "challenging behaviour", the care agency give notice without getting to the root cause of the behaviour or trying to work with the service user and their family'.
Social Worker, community

Other respondents questioned whether some of their care environments gave rise to distressed behaviours, perhaps even being unsuitable for people with dementia, impacting on their behaviours day to day. It was also felt that these behaviours also had other negative impacts, such as making it difficult to find care placements, often resulting in increased lengths of stay, especially in acute hospitals.

Balancing risk/positive risk management

Risk, its assessment and management were issues that were mentioned several times with respondents often struggling to help families to understand and manage risks. This included weighing up the risks and benefits of certain care approaches, and of risks posed in different care settings, for example managing unsafe walking in a hospice environment. Low staffing levels in acute hospital wards and their impact on being able to manage certain risks was also cited:

> 'Patients with dementia have poor awareness of risk and issues relating to their safety in between care visits/overnight. Particularly issues with family's perception of this risk and thinking that all people with dementia are unsafe to be alone and likely need to go into placement'.
> Physiotherapist, acute care

Working with family carers

Respondents talked about their lack of confidence in engaging with family carers and in managing their expectations when supporting the person with dementia, and how this often led to them holding difficult conversations when communicating this to family carers:

> 'Families' expectations – expecting to see their loved ones get better when in reality we look after them till they pass away'.
> Nurse, hospice setting

There were also difficulties reported when there were changes in the person's presenting symptoms and how to engage in communication with family carers about this, for example when goals of care needed to change:

> 'Explaining [swallowing difficulties] to family members/carers...why the patient needs texture modified diet/fluids... Some family members find it difficult to accept'.
> Speech and Language Therapist, acute care

Many understood that engaging other services to support continuity of care was a particular challenge for family carers:

> 'Biggest problems tend to be in joined up communication between health and social services and patients/carers actually being able to

get hold of staff to assist and facilitate signposting to correct agencies'.
Nurse, community

Again, respondents felt the pandemic had negatively impacted on family carers, and described difficulties arising where services had not allowed family carers to accompany the person with dementia to appointments and during hospitalization due to a ban on visiting. It was also acknowledged that these restrictions due to COVID-19 had increased the stress and burden of many family carers.

'Since the pandemic greater challenges in accessing support for carers as no respite, no day care services and unclear if some of these supports will be reinstated. Carer burden has increased exponentially'.
Dementia Link Worker

Some respondents were family carers themselves for a relative with dementia, and identified emotional difficulties when then professionally caring for people with dementia:

'When you are aware of the path dementia progresses on! When it personally affects you, it becomes difficult!'
Professional Carer, social care

CONCLUSION

The combination of the Helpline and survey data has allowed us to form a picture of the most common issues and challenges faced by generalist health and social care practitioners when they work with families affected by dementia. The themes arising from the data have directly informed the structure of the book and the content covered in each chapter. This has allowed us to create a resource that advises on the real-world challenges faced in day-to-day practice, and that will help families affected by dementia as they navigate the complex health and social care landscape.

SOURCES OF SUPPORT

If you have any questions about helping a person with any aspect of dementia, call our free Helpline on 0800 888 6678 or email at helpline@dementiauk.org
If you would prefer a pre-booked appointment by phone or video, call via the Dementia UK website: www.dementiauk.org

REFERENCES

Braun, V. & Clarke, V. (2022) *Thematic analysis: A practical guide.* London: Sage Publications.

Department of Health (DH) (2015) *Prime Minister's challenge on dementia 2020.* London: Department of Health.

Harrison Dening, K., Aldridge, Z. & Hayo, H. (2022) Admiral Nursing: Supporting generalist nurses to work with families affected by dementia. *Nursing Standard.* https://doi:10.7748/ns.2022.e12006

Harrison Dening, K., Hayo, H. & Reddell, C. (Eds.) (2022) *What you really want to know about life with dementia.* London: Jessica Kingsley Publishers.

Parveen, S., Smith, S.J., Sass, C. et al. (2021) Impact of dementia education and training on health and social care staff knowledge, attitudes and confidence: A cross-sectional study. *BMJ Open.* 11(1): e039939. https://doi:10.1136/bmjopen-2020-039939

CHAPTER 2

Recognizing the early symptoms of dementia

THE BENEFITS OF CONTINUITY OF CARE

INTRODUCTION

People are living longer but not necessarily in good health because there has also been an increase in the number who are living with long-term conditions. These conditions require ongoing involvement from health and social care teams, sometimes over many years. The ongoing involvement can lead to the development of a relationship and partnership between the health and social care worker and the person who has the long-term condition(s). Early cognitive changes can often be identified by the health and social care professional which enables a supportive discussion to take place with an appropriate referral for assessment, diagnosis, treatment and planning for the future.

The case study below provides an example of how Liz, a podiatrist, recognized behavioural and cognitive changes in a person who attended her clinic that could be suggestive of dementia, and then what she did because of her concerns. Following the case study, a specialist dementia nurse (Admiral Nurse) writes about what health and social care professionals can do if they are concerned about a person's cognition and behaviour. The Admiral Nurse will also describe the process of dementia screening in primary care and what happens when dementia is suspected.

Liz Watret, Podiatrist

I am a podiatrist, and my story is about continuity of care and how this enables me to observe for changes in our patients over time as we may see some for many years. We are perhaps in the fortunate position that we can build a relationship over time, often discussing major life events, both sad and happy. I am often both surprised and honoured at what people feel they can share with us, especially as someone might attend only a few times a year for basic foot care.

I have worked for nearly 40 years as a podiatrist and feel we are in an ideal position to look for any cognitive changes in our patients, of whom over 50% are over the age of 65 years. We have time to listen whilst we undertake our podiatry interventions. Also, as we attend their feet, they are a captive audience. Conversation length is dictated by the procedure, or the nature of the foot care required, so can be as short as 20 minutes, but sometimes it can be as long as an hour. This amount of time provides an ideal opportunity for noticing changes in personality or cognition. There have been occasions where I have been concerned that a patient is presenting with some changes to their memory and recall, and I will start by sensitively discussing this with them, but on occasions have gone on to discuss such concerns with others. This may be with a family member or health professional, such as their GP, mostly with the person's consent, unless I felt there were concerns of safety of the person or others.

Early in my career there was one lady (let's call her 'Edith') who seemed to be having problems with her memory. I had met Edith only once or twice for basic podiatry treatment. She turned up at the clinic on another occasion, but I did not have her down in the diary for an appointment; she had seemingly attended on the wrong day. I was not expecting her and said as much; perhaps due to my inexperience I did not communicate with her very well. At the time the waiting room was very full and there was another person eagerly waiting for the next appointment, so instead of a conversation where we could have looked at the diary together and resolved the problem, I simply told her she did not have an appointment. The lady was obviously flustered and became very defensive and started to shout, stating that it was my fault, and it must have been me who had made a mistake, not her, and stormed out of the building.

32

However, Edith subsequently called the receptionist to make another appointment saying that she had missed an appointment and could she make another. At the next appointment Edith made no reference to the previous incident. Over the next few visits there were sometimes parts of the conversation that did not always make sense, such as when she said she had to get back home to her parents, and I made notes to this effect in her records. Over the following year, the mistakes in her attendance at the agreed dates and times of appointments became more frequent, and on at least two of these occasions Edith again became defensive and argumentative when I or the receptionist made attempts to discuss this with her. In addition to these occasions, Edith would often present herself at the clinic outside of her next appointment, to check when the next one was. It was following one of these occasions, where Edith became angry, that I asked one of my surgery nursing team colleagues if she knew of the patient. They said they had not seen her in the surgery recently but had known Edith for many years and felt the behaviour I described was out of character.

At Edith's next appointment I took time to ask how she was feeling and managing at home in more depth than I would have done in making basic conversation during a podiatry treatment. Edith shared some of the fears she had about not always remembering things as sharply as she used to; she was very repetitive at times and seemed to forget she had told me some things, only to do so again. I asked if she would be happy if I shared her fears about her memory with her GP, and she agreed. I asked the receptionist to make her a GP appointment and wrote a short note explaining my concerns in our shared records system to give the GP some context to the appointment. About six months after the appointment with her GP, Edith was diagnosed with dementia.

Beth Goss-Hill, Deputy Head of the Admiral Nurse Academy

THE PATHWAY TO DEMENTIA DIAGNOSIS

At some point in life, we all experience memory lapses, like being unable to locate the car keys or recalling a person's name. This can be frustrating but can often be down to tiredness, lack of concentration, stress, ill health or a change in medication. These lapses are usually transient and do not affect everyday living. If these lapses are more frequent and there are other cognitive or behaviour changes this can be more concerning and may need further investigation.

Although, memory loss is the most common symptom experienced by people in the early stages of dementia, it is also important to highlight that there are other cognitive deficits and functional impairments that can be experienced. For some forms of dementia, the person may not have any problems with their memory at all but experience changes in their personality, behaviour, mood and social functioning. In the case study Liz noticed that Edith was exhibiting changes to memory, communication and behaviour, and these were getting increasingly worse over time and affecting her everyday living ability. Table 2.1 lists some of the symptoms that may be experienced by people in the early stages of dementia.

In early-stage dementia the symptoms identified in Table 2.1 are often not in isolation of each other and are not just one-off occurrences but ongoing, causing everyday tasks to become challenging and increasing the risk of additional frustration, anxiety and distress for the symptomatic person and their family.

In the case study of Edith some of these changes were displayed, i.e., difficulties with memory, concentration, communication, planning, mood and behaviour changes. Liz correctly identified that this was out of keeping with how Edith was previously and could identify that these issues were getting worse over time.

When a person experiences the changes suggestive of early-stage dementia they may not understand what is happening, may be concerned and worry about this and seek reasons for why they are experiencing these difficulties. In the case of Edith when she mistakenly turned up for the podiatrist appointment, she did not accept it was her error and the way she was told may have made her feel very vulnerable, hence why she expressed her displeasure.

Table 2.1: Symptoms of early-stage dementia (adapted from Aldridge and Harrison Dening 2019)

Memory and concentration	The most common symptom for most forms of dementia is characterized by short-term and working memory issues whilst leaving the long-term memory relatively intact. There may be frequent repetition of stories, conversation or tasks with little recognition that it has been said before. In frontotemporal dementia (FTD) the memory may be unchanged, but concentration may be affected.
Mood changes	Increasing agitation, anxiety or depression, especially if there is some degree of insight into the changes they are experiencing.
Planning, problem solving and decision making	Everyday tasks that require planning may become more difficult, e.g., cooking, managing finances, keeping appointments. The person may make decisions that are different than before, and this could lead to financial or lifestyle difficulties. Problems with planning, problem solving, and decision making are more common in people who have changes to the frontal lobes of the brain, e.g., FTD and vascular dementia.
Language and communication	Word-finding difficulties, repetitive questioning and difficulty keeping track and responding to conversations can be an issue for people in the early stages of dementia and may be a particular problem for people with FTD and vascular dementia.
Getting lost and misplacing things	Particularly getting lost when in unfamiliar places but can also occur in places that are more familiar due to lack of recognition of visual cues. Problems judging distance and hazards can also lead to more trips, falls or accidents and affect driving ability.
Personality and behaviour changes	The changes to personality and behaviour tend to be less noticeable in most forms of dementia, but in dementias that affect the frontal lobe, e.g., FTD and vascular dementia, these changes can be more problematic in the early stages.

This worry about the changes and what they mean can result in people being reluctant to attend a GP appointment as they may fear getting a diagnosis of dementia and what that could mean for them. Liz had a conversation with Edith about these difficulties and was able to gain her consent to make a GP appointment.

There are other conditions that can mimic the symptoms of

dementia, so it is particularly important that anyone with any of the symptoms identified in Table 2.1 makes an appointment with the GP to have these other health conditions (Table 2.2) identified and treated or ruled out.

Table 2.2: Other conditions that may mimic the symptoms of dementia

Hypothyroidism	This can present as memory difficulties and low mood.
Delirium	This can present as either hyper- or hypoactive delirium leading to decreased cognitive functioning, agitation and restlessness and disorientation to time and place. Apathy, as in hypoactive delirium, can be mistaken for progressive symptoms of dementia.
Infection	Can present with the same features as delirium; most common infections are urinary tract or pneumonia.
Anxiety/depression	Could lead to withdrawal from usual social and day-to-day activities. The concentration and motivation problems caused by anxiety and depression could lead to lower scores in the cognitive examination.
Vascular disease	Such as stroke, heart failure or peripheral vascular disease can lower cognitive functioning and give an increased risk of transient ischaemic attacks.
Vitamin deficiencies – B12 and folate	Can lead to memory disturbances and increased confusion.
Kidney/liver function	Requires blood tests to exclude electrolyte disturbances. Symptoms may include disorientation, confusion, reduced concentration and sleepiness.
Diabetes (hyper-/ hypoglycaemia)	To exclude symptoms of unstable blood glucose levels such as in hyper- or hypoglycaemia which may present as increased confusion and drowsiness and difficulty with coordination. An HbA1c above 87 mmol/mol increases the risk of dementia.
Polypharmacy	Medication may lead to reduced ability to carry out day-to-day tasks, increased falls and cognitive impairment.

All these potential health problems can be treated and or controlled to reduce and even resolve symptoms, should these be the primary cause. These tests should be completed by the GP before any referrals are made to the memory assessment service. If these tests do not indicate any abnormalities, and the cognitive and behavioural symptoms continue to cause concern, the GP should start the process of cognitive assessment.

Cognitive screening tools

Following an initial GP consultation, and where other conditions have been ruled out or effectively treated, the dementia assessment can begin with the patient's consent. The GP or a specialist nurse will take a history of symptoms along with an assessment of cognition using a validated evidence-based brief screening tool. The most common is the General Practitioner Assessment of Cognition (GPCOG) (Brodaty et al. 2002). The GPCOG is designed for use in primary care and has a section that the GP asks the patient to complete and if the score is low there is another section for an informant (usually a family member) to complete. This assessment does not diagnose dementia but can indicate whether further cognitive assessment is required and guide the GP as to whether to refer to a specialist memory assessment service for a more detailed and comprehensive assessment.

A cognitive assessment should include the perspectives of the person with suspected dementia and someone that knows them well, such as a family member or friend. It is important to recognize the valued contribution of family members or supporters who will be able to provide a valuable history around the symptom presentation and progression to support health professionals with their assessments. This is helpful in situations where the person undergoing assessment for dementia is unable to provide a detailed history of their pre-morbid cognition and function, and when changes were initially observed (Fitzpatrick et al. 2020).

If the results of all the tests indicate that there is a possibility that the person may have dementia the GP will refer them to a specialist memory assessment service for further detailed tests to establish their cognitive and everyday living abilities. Alongside cognitive testing a brain scan is often used as a part of the wider assessment of dementia and to rule out potentially treatable changes in the brain, e.g., brain tumours. MRI (magnetic resonance imaging) scans may be requested to help confirm the diagnosis and type of dementia, to identify blood vessel damage and areas of atrophy. CT (computerized tomography) scans are helpful to identify signs of a stroke or a brain tumour. A SPECT (single photon emission computed tomography) scan may be requested which can be helpful in detecting altered blood flow in the brain in more detail than in other forms of scanning (NHS 2022).

In the case study Liz doesn't mention whether Edith lives with anyone or has a family; if she did it would be important that, with Edith's consent, they are fully involved in the assessment process. Family carers should be embraced as partners in care and treatment within the context of a three-way relationship between the person with dementia and the health and social care team (Aldridge and Harrison Dening 2019; Harrison Dening 2019; NICE 2018). Throughout the diagnostic process it is essential to acknowledge the carer as a partner, as they may often be the first person to notice early changes in the person and they can support with the collection of information during the assessment process, so an accurate diagnosis is given. However, this can be complex when circumstances have become chaotic, carers neglect their own needs, and health and social care professionals are limited to short appointments to address one specific problem (Goss-Hill and Aldridge 2020).

Once all assessments have been completed, which include assessment of cognitive deficits, any functional impairment, along with the history of presenting symptoms and the scan results, these will be considered to support a diagnosis to be made by an appropriately trained health professional (NICE 2018). Once a diagnosis has been identified this is then sensitively explained and explored with the patient and their family with time to answer any questions and identify treatments available and support going forward. It is imperative at this point that access to valuable sources of psychological, emotional, physical and social post-diagnostic support are readily available to help the family adjust, gain a better understanding of the symptoms experienced and come to terms with dementia, supporting them to live better with the condition as it progresses. An early diagnosis also allows the whole family to adjust, gain a better understanding and plan ahead to support living as well as possible with dementia and potentially manage other co-morbidities more effectively. Plans can include:

- initiating a Lasting Power of Attorney (health and welfare, and finance)

- discussing future wishes including advance care planning

- accessing financial support
- making adaptions in the home to support independence
- accessing employer support
- arranging reviews
- considering how to cope if emergency care or a hospital admission is needed
- access to post-diagnostic support.

It may be that as symptoms of dementia progress over time, needs also change, requiring specific services and support to dip in and out in a meaningful and appropriate way.

Not having an accurate diagnosis can reduce opportunities to access appropriate treatment and support (Gove et al. 2015; Perry-Young et al. 2018). The benefits that can be gained through accessing the right support and treatment at the right time can enable symptom management, lead to greater understanding of the person and family and facilitate the development of coping strategies to improve quality of life for all parties.

CONCLUSION

This chapter identified how Liz, a podiatrist, observed changes in Edith's cognition and behaviour over time whilst she was engaging in ongoing podiatry treatment. As Liz was concerned, she spoke with Edith about how she felt and was managing at home. This gave Edith the opportunity to talk about her worries regarding her memory. From this conversation Liz was able to seek agreement from Edith to make a GP appointment to have this investigated further. The Admiral Nurse went on to describe the process that takes place regarding cognitive assessment and eventual diagnosis. Once a person is diagnosed with dementia they and their family can then plan for the future, develop coping strategies, and access advice and support so they can live as well as possible with dementia.

SOURCES OF SUPPORT

If you have any questions about helping a person with any aspect of dementia, call our free Helpline on 0800 888 6678 or email at helpline@dementiauk.org
If you would prefer a pre-booked appointment by phone or video, call via the Dementia UK website: www.dementiauk.org

RESOURCES

Dementia UK. **How to get a diagnosis of dementia.** www.dementiauk.org/
information-and-support/specialist-diagnosis-and-support/how-to-get-a-diagnosis-of-dementia

Dementia UK. **After a diagnosis check list.** www.dementiauk.org/get-support/
diagnosis-and-specialist-suppport/after-a-diagnosis-of-dementia-next-steps-checklist

REFERENCES

Aldridge, Z. & Harrison Dening, K. (2019) Improving diagnosis of dementia – The role of the practice nurse. *Practice Nurse.* 49(3): 24–30.

Brodaty, H., Pond, D., Kemp, N.M. et al. (2002) The GPCOG: A new screening test for dementia designed for general practice. *Journal of American Geriatrics Society.* 50(3): 530–534.

Fitzpatrick, D., Doyle, K., Finn, G. et al. (2020) The collateral history: An overlooked core clinical skill. *European Geriatric Medicine.* 11(6): 1003–1007.

Goss-Hill, B. & Aldridge, Z. (2020) Admiral Nursing case management in primary care. *Practice Nurse.* 50(10): 12–17.

Gove, D., Downs, M., Vernooij-Dassen, M. et al. (2015) Stigma and GPs' perceptions of dementia. *Aging & Mental Health.* 20(4): 391–400.

Harrison Dening, K. (2019) Recognition and assessment of dementia in primary care. *British Journal of Community Nursing.* 24(8): 383–387.

National Institute for Health & Care Excellence (NICE) (2018) *Dementia: Assessment, management and support for people living with dementia and their carers (Guideline 97).* www.nice.org.uk/guidance/ng97

NHS (2022) *Tests for diagnosing dementia.* www.nhs.uk/conditions/dementia/diagnosis-tests

Perry-Young, L., Owen, G., Kelly, S. & Owens, C. (2018) How people come to recognise a problem and seek medical help for a person showing early signs of dementia: A systematic review and meta-ethnography. *Dementia.* 17(1): 34–60. doi:10.1177/1471301215626889

CHAPTER 3

There isn't going to
be a happy ending

TRUTH TELLING OR THERAPEUTIC LYING?

INTRODUCTION

For some people who live with a diagnosis of dementia there is a lack of awareness of how the condition affects them, and the changes that it makes to their everyday living abilities. This can adversely affect the support they will accept to enable them to live as well as possible with the diagnosis. This in turn can also negatively affect the life of the person who is providing them with care and support.

The case study below provides an example of the difficulties that can be experienced when a person with dementia has limited awareness of the effects their condition has on them and others. Joanne, a social worker, describes how she attempted to support both the person with dementia and their carer so that both of their needs could be addressed. Following the case study, a specialist dementia nurse (Admiral Nurse) writes about mental capacity and best interest decisions and how this can be implemented in practice. The Admiral Nurse will also explore what to do when there is conflict between a person with dementia and their carer over what is needed.

Often health and social care professionals are concerned about the use of deceptive practices, truth telling and therapeutic lying in people with dementia, and are unclear of when and how this can be used effectively. The Admiral Nurse will explore this approach and how and when it might be appropriate to use it.

Joanne Bush, Social Worker

As a newly qualified social worker I supported a carer, Sue, who was finding it difficult to support her partner, Bill. The couple had met ten years previously when they had both moved to independent living retirement flats in the same complex. Four years prior to this, Bill had been diagnosed with dementia and, over time, his needs had progressively increased, with much of his care falling to Sue. Bill could no longer make his own meals or drinks, and often needed support to wash and dress. He had become disorientated as to night and day and would regularly knock on Sue's door throughout the night, seemingly feeling insecure when Sue was not with him. Bill had little awareness of his increasing dependency on Sue, proclaiming an ability to not only meet all of his own needs, but also to work full time in a sales role, even though he had long since retired. Bill would regularly walk around the apartment carrying a briefcase and talk about business he had to be getting on with. Sue was clearly exhausted and expressed a desire to engage in social activities without having to worry about him. Bill did not understand why Sue needed this and, in conversation with me, became agitated and was adamant Sue's concerns were unfounded.

I completed a mental capacity assessment of Bill's ability to make a decision about his care needs and felt he was not able to weigh up the information needed to make a decision. I explored whether home care or day care were viable options but as Bill did not acknowledge he had any needs, they were not.

Over a period of several weeks, we progressively ran out of options to explore, and it became clear that Sue could not carry on caring for Bill and she would often leave me exasperated voicemails stating that something urgently needed to change. With the input of Sue, I made the best interest decision that Bill would have to move to residential accommodation more suitable to his level of need. However, given that Bill did not accept these needs, it was not easy to convince him to go willingly to a care home. So, after a suitable home was selected, we decided the only way was to use deceptive methods to get him there.

Bill went willingly there with Sue, and they sat in the communal area and once settled, Sue then left without telling Bill she was going. I remained at the home with Bill to support him and to explain to him why he was there. However, in Bill's eyes he was a man who thought he went out to work daily and was perfectly capable of meeting his own needs. Trying to explain to Bill that he was now going to stay at the care home was one of the most difficult times of my career. Bill did not take the news well and after shouting at staff to get the police, he tried to break through the glass door at the entrance to escape. The police were called, and Bill ended up being sectioned under the Mental Health Act in a mental health ward.

I was asked to attend a tribunal a week later and saw Bill. I have never seen someone age so much in such a short space of time and that image of him remains with me. Bill was later transferred to a more secure home that could meet his needs.

As a more experienced social worker, I look back at this case and can see several things I would have approached differently. I was trying to consider both Bill and Sue's conflicting needs and therefore could not be in a position to fully support both. With hindsight there are many things I would have done differently. Not least, I would have been open about the emotional impact the case was having on me and would have explored ways of managing this more thoroughly. However, I recognize that the outcome is unlikely to have been any different as Bill's perception of his life was based on a reality that did not exist. Bill wanted to go to work and come home and be with Sue. He had no awareness of the cost to Sue's health and wellbeing whilst she tried to support him, and if he did know this, he may have chosen a different option.

In these types of situations there is not going to be a happy ending, but there are better and worse ways of navigating the potential pitfalls to ensure the needs of all involved are met and emotional resilience is developed.

Lucy Chamberlain, Admiral Nurse Practitioner

Dementia is a condition that affects not only the person with the diagnosis, but also the people around them who are involved in that person's life. Inevitably, the greatest effect will be upon the person closest to the person with dementia, as seen here in the case of Bill and Sue. Joanne identified the impact of the changes in Bill on his care partner, Sue, affecting her sleep, ability to function in life outside the home and the increased level of help she needed to provide to Bill. Joanne had explored solutions that could support Sue in her caring role but felt Bill's lack of insight into his situation made plans difficult to put in place.

'Carer burnout' is a widely recognized and common outcome of caring for someone with dementia (Hazzan et al. 2022), and a significant factor in precipitating the move of a person with dementia into residential care as their needs increase (Young et al. 2021). Bill's needs had moved beyond that which could be managed at home by a family carer, and so the decision was taken that it was in Bill's 'best interests' for him to move into residential care.

CAPACITY AND BEST INTERESTS

The Mental Capacity Act 2005 (MCA) is designed to empower and protect the rights of people who lack 'mental capacity' – a legal concept that refers to someone's ability to make decisions about aspects of their life, including care and treatment. According to the MCA (2005):

> a person lacks capacity in relation to a matter if at the material time he is unable to make a decision for himself in relation to the matter because of an impairment of, or a disturbance in the functioning of, the mind or brain.

To have capacity, a person must be able to:

- understand the information relevant to the decision they are making

- retain that information for long enough to make the decision

- weigh up the information as part of their decision-making process

- communicate that decision to others.

The MCA (2005, s1, 1–6) has five core principles that protect the rights of people who lack capacity to make their own decisions, and these must underpin the actions of all professionals involved in the care and treatment of people with dementia:

1. A person must be assumed to have capacity unless it is established that he lacks capacity.

2. A person is not to be treated as unable to make a decision unless all practicable steps to help him to do so have been taken without success.

3. A person is not to be treated as unable to make a decision merely because he makes an unwise decision.

4. An act done, or decision made, under this Act for or on behalf of a person who lacks capacity must be done, or made, in his best interests.

5. Before the act is done, or the decision is made, regard must be had to whether the purpose for which it is needed can be as effectively achieved in a way that is less restrictive of the person's rights and freedom of action.

When decisions need to be made in a person's best interests, the Act directs that the person/people making the determination must consider '*all the relevant circumstances*', and outlines steps the decision maker(s) must take to include the person with the diagnosis of dementia in the process, and/or to ascertain the person's relevant prior wishes, preferences and feelings and to include those involved in the person's care.

It is also important to note that capacity assessments are 'time and decision specific' – that is that they only cover the decision that needs answering at the time it is asked; there is no blanket capacity assessment that covers all that person's decisions.

In practice, this means that although only one professional – Joanne – might need the answer to a decision that needs making, they must speak with all other relevant people involved in that person's – Bill's – life. This might be family members, friends, other professionals, and should include anyone who has been closely involved with Bill and Sue. Joanne would need to give Bill plenty of time to assess his capacity, making sure as much as possible is done to help him take in what is being discussed, and taking his expressed wishes into account, both now and any known from the past when he may have discussed a similar situation.

Bill's dementia had impaired his ability to understand his care needs and situation. His 'reality' was as real to him as ours is to us, and therefore trying to persuade, reason or explain the situation, as experienced by Sue, to him would be extremely difficult and challenging for Bill, and as Joanne discovered, could lead to Bill becoming agitated and angry.

In considering the possible options, Joanne decided not to try home or day care due to Bill's likely refusal and distressed response. However, it could be argued that it may have been worth trying this first as a 'least restrictive alternative' that could possibly have delayed any move into care. It is difficult to introduce home or day care as an intervention to people who see no need for it, but not impossible. This can be where the boundaries between truth telling and lying can become blurred and can cause anxiety and discomfort for both family carers and professionals.

THERAPEUTIC LYING

A person with dementia can become confused with memories from an earlier period in their life, and these memories become the person's present-day reality (Casey et al. 2020). James and Caiazza (2018) found that 'therapeutic lying' can be beneficial where the person with dementia does not share the same reality as the carer, used as part of a person-centred approach and implemented in a way that is sympathetic to the needs and treatment goals of the person with dementia. Lies and deception are widely used where it is felt that the truth may be harmful or distressing to a person with dementia (Jackman 2020; Mills et al. 2019). For example, someone who believes a long deceased loved one to be still alive could be 're-bereaved' each time they are told that the person is dead. It is perhaps kinder and in their best interests to fabricate a 'story' (therapeutic lie) that makes more sense in that person's reality, for example that their loved one is at work or on holiday. Perhaps Bill may have accepted a sitting service at home if he believed that the person was a trainee employee he was supervising?

The concept of such 'stories' can help carers and professionals to engage with people with dementia in a way that promotes the person-centred aim underlying a 'story' (in this case perhaps a story supporting Bill to remain at home by giving Sue a break) with the least distress to all involved. Family carers have often based their whole relationship or self-image on being honest and open with their loved one and so may need support and time to understand how to change this habit of a lifetime. It can be helpful to look at the language we use in these circumstances and explain to them that 'truth' and 'lie' are value-laden terms. These are often not binary or no longer as straightforward and helpful, so it can often be helpful for them to explore the different reality that someone with dementia may be inhabiting and how they can join them there with stories, rather than try to drag them out into our reality.

For example, maybe Bill would have come to accept day care if he attended a few times with Sue, being told the 'story' that it was more a social setting, such as a café that they both enjoyed. Over time Sue may have then started withdrawing for short periods to 'pick up shopping' until Bill became settled and more familiar with the day care setting. This could have the long-term goal of allowing Bill to get used to communal settings, and being apart from Sue, which may have made the transition to permanent care less jarring for him.

When the time came for Bill to move to a care home, it may have been easier for Bill to accept a 'story' that fitted his self-image of a man who had no needs and still worked. Such a story could perhaps be a holiday, working away or staying here (in the care setting) temporarily whilst disruptive work was being done on the house or Sue was away visiting family. Confronting Bill with the inexplicable information that he has been placed in a care home and that Sue has gone home and left him there could lead to feelings of abandonment, panic and fear, which then understandably led to him shouting for help and trying to find a way out.

MULTI-DISCIPLINARY WORKING

Telling the truth is a key tenet of health and social care, as are valuing a person's autonomy and bodily integrity. Going against this, no matter how compassionately motivated, can cause tension with core personal and professional values (Dresser 2021) which can be hard to reconcile. Utilizing a multi-disciplinary approach to the best interest decision-making process can be protective emotionally and practically for the professional, the person with dementia and their carer, sharing the decision-making burden across all the relevant people involved. This may include district nurses, GPs, social workers, specialists, such as memory services and Admiral Nurses, as well as wider family members. Bringing other professionals on board may also open up a wider menu of options that the decision maker may not have been aware of, such as medication, carer educational courses and so forth, or enable a discussion about what level of care Bill needed and whether the proposed care home would be suitable to meet those needs.

Best interest decisions should take in a wide range of factors which include 'the views of...anyone engaging in caring for the person' (S.4, 7(b)). The use of an advocate or independent mental capacity advocate (IMCA) for the person with dementia if they are unable to participate themselves is particularly valuable. In a case such as Bill and Sue's, an IMCA will focus solely on Bill's needs, which may not necessarily align with Sue's. Research shows that carers find the experience of having to make such huge decisions for the person they care for, such as a move into a residential care service, distressing (Carter et al. 2018).There can be deep regret and feelings of guilt if this does not run smoothly, further highlighting the usefulness to Bill and Sue of having an IMCA involved to advocate for his needs.

CONFLICTING NEEDS BETWEEN A CARER AND PERSON WITH DEMENTIA

Harrison Dening and Aldridge (2019) identify that relationships in dementia care need to delicately balance the interests between the different people involved. In practice, there is sometimes an imbalance between the weight given to the perspectives and wishes of the person with dementia and those of the carer. In the case outlined, Bill wants to stay at home and doesn't feel there is a problem at all as he lacks insight, yet Sue is increasingly unable to meet his significant and growing care needs and is repeatedly asking for help. Remaining objective in the face of carer distress is not easy, and professionals can find themselves automatically 'siding' one way or another.

Similarly, beliefs or service imperatives that 'the best place for someone with dementia is at home' can blinker professionals, and the drive to keep people at home at all costs and may inadvertently result in the deterioration of the carer's emotional and physical wellbeing.

CLINICAL SUPERVISION

Joanne reflected on the emotional impact this case had on her. The use of clinical supervision for health and social care professionals is widely acknowledged to be supportive of them, improves patient safety and care and promotes professional development (Snowden et al. 2020). Admiral Nurses access monthly supervision facilitated by practice and professional development specialists at Dementia UK, which provides a safe space for self-care, promotes resilience, supports learning and enables time to explore complex cases with peers (Russell et al. 2022). As a professional, it is invaluable to be able to share these emotionally laden cases that challenge our professional and personal values, and to explore what went well, and what could improve for next time, as well as allow ourselves to be challenged as to our actions and their underlying reasoning.

CONCLUSION

This chapter explored how social worker Joanne experienced the competing needs and wishes of a couple, where the carer, Sue, was struggling to cope with Bill's growing and changing care needs. Because of his dementia, Bill lacked insight into those needs, and was unable to take part in planning his own care. The resultant care home placement broke down leading to hospital admission. Joanne felt she could have done things differently, although Bill's needs would always have led to care placement. The Admiral Nurse explored the underlying legal framework of capacity assessments and best interest decisions and discussed the concept of therapeutic lying in the context of dementia care, identifying ways to support professionals in navigating this.

SOURCES OF SUPPORT

If you have any questions about helping a person with any aspect of dementia, call our free Helpline on 0800 888 6678 or email at helpline@dementiauk.org

If you would prefer a pre-booked appointment by phone or video, call via the Dementia UK website: www.dementiauk.org

RESOURCES

Mental Capacity Act Code of Practice. www.gov.uk/government/publications/ mental-capacity-act-code-of-practice

Social Care Institute for Excellence: Mental capacity in practice. www.scie.org. uk/mca/practice

What is truth? An inquiry about truth and lying in dementia care. Mental Health Foundation. www.mentalhealth.org.uk/sites/default/files/2022-09/ MHF-dementia-truth-inquiry-report.pdf

REFERENCES

Carter, G., McLaughlin, D., Kernohan, W.G. et al. (2018) The experiences and preparedness of family carers for best interest decision-making of a relative living with advanced dementia: A qualitative study. *Journal of Advanced Nursing.* 74(7): 1595–1604.

Casey, D., Lynch, U., Murphy, K. et al. (2020) Telling a 'good or white lie': The views of people living with dementia and their carers. *Dementia.* 19(8): 2582–2600.

Dresser, R. (2021) A tangled web: Deception in everyday dementia care. *The Journal of Law, Medicine & Ethics.* 49(2): 257–262.

Harrison Dening, K. & Aldridge, Z. (2019) Admiral Nurse case management: A model of caregiver support for families affected by dementia. *OBM Geriatrics.* 3(2): 53. https://doi:10.21926/obm.geriatr.1902053

Hazzan, A.A., Dauenhauer, J., Follansbee, P. et al. (2022) Family caregiver quality of life and the care provided to older people living with dementia: Qualitative analyses of caregiver interviews. *BMC Geriatrics.* 22: 86. https://doi. org/10.1186/s12877-022-027870

Jackman, L. (2020) Extending the Newcastle Model: How therapeutic communication can reduce distress in people with dementia. *Nursing Older People.* doi:0.7748/nop.2020.e1206

James, I. & Caiazza, R. (2018) Therapeutic lies in dementia care: Should psychologists teach others to be person-centred liars? *Behavioural and Cognitive Psychotherapy.* 46(4): 454–462.

Mental Capacity Act (2005) www.legislation.gov.uk/ukpga/2005/9/introduction

Mills, R., Jackman, L., Mahesh, M. et al. (2019) Key dimensions of therapeutic lies in dementia care: A new taxonomy. *OBM Geriatrics.* 3(1): 32. https://doi:10.21926/ obm.geriatr.1901032

Russell, S., Daly, R., Dodds, P. et al. (2022) Using online practice action learning sets for clinical supervision. *Nursing Times.* 118: 5. www.nursingtimes.net/ clinical-archive/clinical-supervision/using-online-practice-action-learning-sets-for-clinical-supervision-11-04-2022

Snowdon, D.A., Sargent, M., Williams, C.M., Maloney, S., Caspers, K. & Taylor, N.F. (2019) Effective clinical supervision of allied health professionals: A mixed methods study. *BMC Health Services Research.* 20(1): 2. doi:10.1186/ s12913-019-4873-8

Young, J.A., Lind, C. & Orange, J. (2021) A qualitative systematic review of experiences of persons with dementia regarding transition to long-term care. *Dementia.* 20(1): 5–27.

CHAPTER 4

Involving people with dementia and their families in research

INTRODUCTION

Being involved in research can make a difference to the lives of people with dementia and their families now and in the future. Whilst a lot of research in dementia is focused on the development of new treatments, it is just as important that research looks at how to improve the care and support of people with dementia and their families who are living with dementia now. Sadly, dementia research doesn't get anywhere near the amount of funding that other health conditions like cancer do, and so the opportunities for people to take part in research are often limited.

Research in dementia has come a long way. Historically, people with dementia were simply not included in research at all – it was thought that they lacked the ability to take part or would not be reliable informants (Wilkinson 2002: 9–25). Thankfully, research now recognizes that people with dementia are experts in their own lives and that the active involvement of people with dementia in all stages of research is vital to ensure research is focused on the things that really matter to them. Some of the most exciting recent innovations in dementia research involve the inclusion of people with dementia as co-researchers (The Dementia Enquirers 2023).

We still have hurdles to overcome in dementia research – the voices of people from minority communities are overlooked and we need to get better at ensuring that people with more advanced dementia are also involved in research.

Sarra Blackman, Research Nurse
Case 1

Working as a research nurse, I was recruiting to a study that involved a trial of a novel medication in the treatment of Alzheimer's dementia. We were approached by a family who wanted to enrol a family member who had a diagnosis of dementia. The family were very passionate about the trial and became very emotional during discussions. As with any research, there are inclusion and exclusion criteria that need to be applied when considering each potential participant to ensure that the study is right for them, and they are a suitable participant for the study.

From what the family said it appeared that this individual would be eligible for the study. I made an appointment to discuss the study, however the person with dementia was not able to understand what the research was about as they no longer had the capacity to do so, despite the family wishing them to be a participant. It was important to explain to the family at this point that it would not be possible to enrol the person into the study as the person with dementia did not have the capacity to make such decisions. This was incredibly distressing for the family as they felt a desperation to get the person with dementia on the medication trial.

Case 2

Working as a research nurse, I was recruiting participants to a study which involved quite lengthy questionnaires. The research team were looking for certain patient populations to join the study including people with Lewy body dementia and Parkinson's dementia. As these diagnoses are rare, we knew that it would be challenging to recruit participants to our study. So, part of my role involved approaching clinicians working in the field to raise the profile of the research study so they could suggest its value to their eligible patients.

However, over time it became more difficult when asking clinicians to identify possible participants from their patient groups. One clinician felt that this study was too onerous and burdensome for this patient population and so had not raised the subject with any of their patients, despite one patient being eligible. As our trust offers research opportunities with an 'opt in' policy it meant that the research team were not able to approach patients directly to offer the opportunity to take part if they had not expressed an interest in hearing about it previously from a member of the clinical team.

However, another member of the clinical team was a research champion and was also working with us to identify potential participants through their clinic lists. Through this role they identified the same patient by running a patient report on their systems. They approached the clinician to discuss the patient's appropriateness to potentially participate. The clinician explained that they did not feel that the patient should be approached giving the reason that he felt the questionnaire was too long. The research champion respectfully challenged the clinician's reasons and promoted the rationale of allowing each patient to make their own choices regarding research participation.

By chance the patient heard about the research through a patient group she attended. She was keen to hear more about the study and requested the participant information sheet to consider the study further. Following ethical protocols, she was given four days to consider the information and encouraged to speak to family and friends about the study. Following this she was keen to participate and was enrolled in the study and continued to support the study for a number of years.

Dr Emma Wolverson, Research Lead, Dementia UK

Research matters to people with dementia and their families. After getting that life-changing diagnosis people with dementia and their families can feel lost and alone. Wendy Mitchell, a research champion diagnosed with young onset dementia, has spoken about how research gave her hope at this difficult time (see the YouTube film of Wendy Mitchell, Research Champion in the Resources section). Research can provide a way to make a difference to the lives of people with dementia now and in the future. Participating in research can be a way for families affected by dementia to feel useful or to give something back to professionals or services who have been supportive.

Research is important for health and social care professionals too, not least because we know that people who are cared for at research-active sites are more likely to experience better outcomes (Jonker et al. 2020). Being involved in research makes staff happier and makes people stay in their jobs longer (Rees and Bracewell 2019). Research also benefits health and social care systems, by ensuring that we continually improve the care that people with dementia and their families receive. Research helps professionals to understand the changing needs of the communities they serve and to ensure they are delivering the care in the best possible way.

In practice, carrying out research involving people with dementia and their families is not always easy and the case studies presented highlight two common issues that impact the delivery of dementia research – issues of consent and research gatekeeping.

INFORMED CONSENT TO TAKE PART IN RESEARCH

Any researcher in dementia who has stood before an ethics committee will tell you that the capacity to give informed consent to research is always of paramount concern. Seeking an individual's consent is a fundamental ethical principle and vital to safeguarding research participants from harm. To give informed consent a person must have the capacity to decide whether to take part in the research, have been properly informed about the research and have agreed to participate without pressure or coercion.

In the UK, in accordance with the Mental Capacity Act (2005) we should always start from the assumption that a person has capacity, and we have a duty to do all we can to support a person's ability to make a decision. Anyone responsible for seeking consent for a research study must be confident in assessing a person's capacity to participate. As people with dementia's abilities may fluctuate, it is vital that consent is assessed as an ongoing process throughout research. Of course, people have the right to change their mind and to withdraw from research, without giving a reason.

To make an informed decision about taking part in research people must understand what taking part will involve. Researchers and clinicians that are supporting recruitment to research must make sure that people are given information about the study in a way that they can understand; this is in the form of a 'participant information sheet'. As researchers it is vital in designing our research procedures, processes and materials that we work with people with dementia and carers as experts by experience. Patient and public involvement groups can advise researchers on everything from making sure information is written in a range of accessible formats, to checking that test procedures are not too demanding or laborious. There are guides written by people with dementia about the best ways to involve people with dementia in research (see The Dementia Enquirers in the Resources section).

Sometimes people may lose capacity during a research project (perhaps if the study has been following people over a long time) and the research will need to have clear procedures in place for what happens to ensure that people are protected. The cohort study Improving the Experience of Dementia and Enhancing Active Life-Living Well with Dementia (IDEAL) (Clare et al. 2014) is one such example, as the study took place over two years. On entry to the study participants had to nominate a personal consultee who would be able to say whether they should continue or not if the person lost capacity.

Research can involve people with dementia without capacity to consent. To do this the research must have clear processes to get consent from someone else, usually a close family member, on the person's behalf. Researchers will ask the person giving consent to think about what the person with dementia's values and beliefs were about research and what they would have thought about the study. Some people with dementia may have advance statements which include their wishes about whether they want to be involved in research.

It is not clear in Case Study 1 whether the study had procedures in place for the person's family to give consent on their relative's behalf. Given the family's disappointment, it would be important to connect them to other opportunities to take part in research. One example might be signposting them to Join Dementia Research, a research register which matches people to studies (see Resources section).

GATEKEEPERS

Gatekeepers are people with power and authority to either admit or refuse researchers access to a particular setting or to potential participants (Sharkey et al. 2010). These are not just service managers but can be health and social care professionals, like those in Case Study

2, who have been asked to recruit people to a study. Family carers, sometimes unintentionally, can also act as gatekeepers.

Gatekeeping is a persistent issue in recruiting to dementia research and often means that sample sizes in studies are much smaller than desired. Gatekeeping is also an ethical issue, because gatekeepers may prevent people from making their own decisions about taking part in research, overriding their autonomy.

So why do health and social professionals act as gatekeepers? Gatekeeping is not necessarily a conscious decision; for some the pressure of a busy caseload and lack of time means that professionals don't feel they have the time to get involved and actively recruit to research. Attitudes and low confidence towards research can also result in gatekeeping. For example, sometimes clinicians don't feel confident in talking about research or in answering questions that arise, so don't share information about studies.

On other occasions people make a conscious decision to be a gatekeeper. Case Study 2 highlights one of the main reasons that professionals decide to withhold research opportunities; a fear of over-burdening the person with dementia or their family carer. People with dementia often don't have ongoing contact or monitoring from healthcare services which limits opportunities to hear about research. Instead, people with dementia and their families typically only encounter health and social care professionals in times of crisis (Alzheimer's Society 2022). Here gatekeepers may feel a need, or responsibility, to protect people who are struggling. This may be particularly true where there is a belief that research exploring sensitive topics might cause distress or where research procedures are perceived as burdensome.

Another common reason for gatekeeping is a reluctance to talk openly to the person and their family about their diagnosis, perhaps because the professional is uncertain if the person is aware or remembers they have a diagnosis of dementia. Studies about palliative and end-of-life care often encounter a lot of gatekeepers because of a reluctance to have conversations about the progressive and terminal nature of dementia and identifying that the person is in the final stages of their illness (Kars et al. 2016).

Doubts about the importance of the quality of the research are further reasons that a gatekeeper might not support research.

Perhaps the gatekeeper doesn't see the value of the topic or the intervention being tested, or perhaps they doubt the study's methods or approach. In my own research, I encountered enormous resistance to advertising a study looking for participants to co-design a website for people with dementia as the healthcare professionals I spoke to strongly believed that people with dementia did not use the internet for support.

So, what can you do as a health or social care professional to ensure that people with dementia and their families have access to research opportunities? How do we ensure that we don't become gatekeepers and what do we do if we encounter others who are gatekeeping?

1. **Be a research champion**

   Both case studies highlight the important role that could be played by research champions in promoting awareness, engagement and delivering research. Research champions help to promote studies, set studies up in services and support participant recruitment. Usually, research champions are given training in research and dedicated time within their role to focus on research. To find out about local opportunities contact your trust's Research and Development Team, your local clinical research network or the National Institute of Health Research (NIHR).

2. **Build your own research confidence and expertise**

   It is vital that health and social care professionals feel confident and knowledgeable when talking about research. Being a regular 'consumer' of research is one way to increase your confidence. Reading research blogs, listening to podcasts, attending webinars and registering for academic journal alerts are all ways for you to engage more with research. NHS trust Research and Development departments often run research training events. Universities also offer research training courses at various levels. Supporting student research projects can also be a great way to get started.

3. **When approached about supporting research – ask questions!**

   If researchers come seeking your support for a study, have your questions ready (see Box 4.1). Remember the most successful studies involve people with dementia, family carers and health and social care professions right from the start when they are designing the study.

Box 4.1: Questions to ask researchers who seek your support in sharing their research

→ How have people with dementia and their families been involved in designing this research?

→ Why is this topic important?

→ Why is this research needed now?

→ How will this topic make a difference to the lives of people with dementia and their families?

→ How will you share the findings of this research with people with dementia and their families?

---

4. **Consider how you can build a research culture**

The sites that are often most successful at getting people involved in research are those in which taking part in research is the norm and where the whole team values and expects to be involved in research. Embedding research in practice takes time (see NIHR 2023), but small things can make a big difference. One example might be simplifying a research process to support health professionals to talk about research – perhaps all clinical appointment letters could include a statement in the footer to indicate that your organization is research active, and that patients or clients may be approached about joining research studies. This immediately helps clinicians feel more confident about sharing research opportunities.

5. **Work with patient research ambassadors**

Patient and public research ambassadors can have an incredible impact with their enthusiasm and passion for research having a strong motivating influence on others. Most NHS trusts and universities will have patient and public research ambassadors who have a lot to say about the value of research. Most research funders now require patient and public involvement in the design and conduct of research studies. Where people with dementia and family carers themselves can explain the value of a study to professionals and to potential participants this should be supported. Imagine the impact in Case Study 1 if the lady who took part in the study became a research champion and came to speak to the clinician about what she got from being involved in research.

CONCLUSION

Research is central to providing better care and support to people with dementia and their families. People with dementia have a right to be involved in research. Health and social care professionals need to feel confident and empowered to be involved in research. Our most important allies in increasing research capacity are people with dementia and their families themselves.

SOURCES OF SUPPORT

If you have any questions about helping a person with any aspect of dementia, call our free Helpline on 0800 888 6678 or email at helpline@dementiauk.org

If you would prefer a pre-booked appointment by phone or video, call via the Dementia UK website: www.dementiauk.org

RESOURCES

Join Dementia Research. www.joindementiaresearch.nihr.ac.uk

Wendy Mitchell, Research Champion – YouTube. Wendy Mitchell shares her dementia journey and explains why encouraging others to take part in dementia research is so important to her. www.youtube.com/watch?v=GKrcbcbpXPA

The Dementia Enquirers. Gold standards for co-research. https://dementiaenquirers.org.uk/wp-content/uploads/2023/02/gold-standard-for-co-research.pdf

REFERENCES

Alzheimer's Society (2022) *Left to cope alone: The unmet support needs after a diagnosis of dementia.* www.alzheimers.org.uk/about-us/policy-and-influencing/left-cope-alone-unmet-support-needs-after-dementia-diagnosis

Clare, L., Nelis, N.M., Quinn, C. et al. (2014) Improving the experience of dementia and enhancing active life – living well with dementia: Study protocol for the IDEAL study. *Health and Quality of Life Outcomes.* 12(1): 1–15.

The Dementia Enquirers (2023) *Gold standards for co-research.* https://dementiaenquirers.org.uk/wp-content/uploads/2023/02/gold-standard-for-co-research.pdf

Jonker, L., Fisher, S.J. & Dagnan, D. (2020) Patients admitted to more research-active hospitals have more confidence in staff and are better informed about their condition and medication: Results from a retrospective cross-sectional study. *Journal of Evaluation in Clinical Practice.* 26(1): 203–208.

Kars, M.C., van Thiel, G.J., van der Graaf, R. et al. (2016) A systematic review of reasons for gatekeeping in palliative care research. *Palliative Medicine.* 30(6): 533–548.

Mental Capacity Act (2005) www.legislation.gov.uk/ukpga/2005/9/introduction

National Institute for Health and Care Research (NIHR) (2023) Embedding a research culture. www.nihr.ac.uk/health-and-care-professionals/engagement-and-participation-in-research/embedding-a-research-culture.htm

Rees, M.R. & Bracewell, M. (2019) Academic factors in medical recruitment: Evidence to support improvements in medical recruitment and retention by improving the academic content in medical posts. *Postgraduate Medical Journal.* 95(1124): 323–327.

Sharkey, K., Savulescu, J., Aranda, S. et al. (2010) Clinician gatekeeping in clinical research is not ethically defensible: An analysis. *Journal of Medical Ethics,* 36(6): 363–366.

Wilkinson, H. (Ed.) (2002) *Including people with dementia in research – The perspectives of people with dementia: Research methods and motivations.* London: Jessica Kingsley Publishers.

CHAPTER 5

Communication and dementia

INTRODUCTION

Difficulties with communication can be a common feature of all types of dementia and may be the first noticeable symptom. Communication difficulties can stem from problems with expression, where people with dementia have problems finding the right words, with fluency and with forming sounds needed to make certain words. There may also be difficulties in understanding verbal communication from others, for example following instructions or engaging in a conversation. Dementia may eventually lead to the complete loss of verbal communication, meaning those around them must rely solely on non-verbal cues to be able to communicate meaningfully.

In some cases, communication can become tangential and repetitive, conversation may become metaphorical and meaning located in the past. The cognitive symptoms of dementia can also impact on communication, for example making it difficult to engage in 'small talk' about their day, especially if they cannot remember what has happened. Symptoms such as false beliefs, hallucinations and delusions can also disrupt communication, as the person may be inhabiting a different reality to those around them, making it hard for them to know how to respond. Professionals have to communicate not only with the person with dementia, but with their family members as well, and this can present a whole host of different challenges. For example, when there are difficult family dynamics at play, or when the emotional and psychological needs of the family carer make it difficult for them to take information about the person with dementia on board.

This chapter uses three vignettes to illustrate some of the most common communication challenges faced by professionals working with families affected by dementia. The cases are drawn from experience working as an Admiral Nurse both in the community and on the Admiral Nurse Dementia Helpline. Inspiration for these case studies has also been taken from the responses to the survey which informed the structure of this book.

Three common challenges to communication
Anira

Anira is 81 and has a diagnosis of Alzheimer's disease. The diagnosis was made five years ago. Anira lived at home with her husband Rohan until a year ago when he made the decision to admit Anira into long-term care as he was struggling to cope. Anira's verbal fluency is affected by dementia making it hard for her to initiate and maintain a conversation. She often struggles to find the right words, and sometimes will unconsciously substitute a different word in place of the one she can't find. Anira is often disorientated, sometimes thinking she is still in her own home, and frequently becomes distressed when she cannot locate her husband. As a result, she is frequently found walking the hallways in the care home in search of him. The following is an example of the dialogue between Anira and a member of the care staff when it is time for tea in the lounge and Anira has been found walking in the hall:

Anira: Ah finally! Can you help me? I can't find Rohan. He said he wouldn't be from…wouldn't… Oh!

Care staff: Hello Anira, I've been looking for you. It's tea-time in the main lounge now, come with me.

Anira: (becoming visibly distressed) But I'm trying… Oh! … I'm trying…

Care staff: (interrupting Anira) Come on, it's this way (puts arm round Anira to gently guide her).

Anira: NO! (pushes nurse's arm away) Where is Rohan!?

In this example communication is clearly difficult for Anira, and a lack of awareness of the right way to support her with her communication difficulty is resulting in her distressed behaviour.

Ahmed

Ahmed has a diagnosis of mixed Alzheimer's and vascular dementia. He lives alone in a small retirement flat, which he moved to some years before his dementia diagnosis. He has recently had a minor fall, sustaining a wound on his leg which needs dressing, so the district nurse team have become involved. The dressing itself is causing no problem, and Ahmed is happy to allow the nurses into the flat to attend to his wound. However, the team have noted that Ahmed often seems preoccupied with perceived problems with his neighbours. He thinks that the residents on his floor are letting in lots of small children, and he reports that he can often hear them through the walls, shouting and laughing. He also tells the nurses that the children have been coming into his flat at night and moving his things around, although he says he has never seen them. The nurses make all the appropriate tests to rule out an infection or other causes of delirium, and so make a referral to the memory service, the outcome of which is that Ahmed is likely misidentifying the sounds of the TV from his immediate neighbours. However, the nurses are struggling to know how to respond to and reassure Ahmed in the moment when he is expressing these beliefs, which feel very real to him.

Anna and Mary

Anna has been caring for her wife, Mary, for almost eight years. During this time, she was diagnosed with Lewy body dementia, and whilst she has experienced numerous falls and infections, she has always recovered. Mary is currently in an acute hospital ward, having had another fall at home, and has been diagnosed with a chest infection. She has been treated with intravenous antibiotics, but the infection is not responding. Mary is now bedbound and is unable to swallow, so there has been a recent assessment by the speech and language therapist. A new nurse has just come on shift to care for Mary and sees in the notes that it has been explained to Anna that Mary is now approaching the end of life.

When the nurse comes to the bedside, she is immediately confronted by Anna who is distraught, feeling that Mary is being denied fluids. She wants to know when they will be putting a feeding tube in and appears to have no understanding that Mary is considered to be approaching the end of life.

(Pseudonyms have been used to ensure anonymity.)

Amy Kerti, Admiral Nurse

Communication challenges are present across all types of dementia, although their exact nature will vary depending on the type and stage of dementia that each individual is experiencing. Dementia can impact communication in a number of different ways, and it is important to be aware of these potential challenges before thinking about how we might support people with dementia in their communication (see Box 5.1).

Box 5.1: Types of communication difficulties experienced by people with dementia

→ difficulty expressing self (expressive aphasia)

→ word-finding difficulties

→ problems with fluency

→ difficulty forming the sounds needed to make certain words

→ difficulties understanding the communication of others (receptive aphasia)

→ difficulties understanding the context of communication

→ repeating self

→ psychological problems affecting communication (e.g., withdrawing due to depression/apathy).

(Adapted from Pepper and Harrison Dening 2023)

As well as the communication difficulties caused directly by the dementia, there may also be social invalidation by others, for example family members may try to protect the person they care for by overcompensating for their memory and recall difficulties, and talking for them. This is typically an act of love but it is sometimes driven by embarrassment. As symptoms advance over time, family members may increasingly try to 'rescue' the person with dementia in social situations, unintentionally causing further invalidation.

PERSON-CENTRED COMMUNICATION

Humans are social animals motivated by validation, acceptance and respect. If these needs are not met, verbal communication and body language is used in an attempt to elicit these expressions from others and the environment. People with dementia can experience social invalidation early in the disease. Kitwood's (1997) model of person-centred care is the dominant model that describes how best to meet the needs of people with dementia. He proposes several core needs: attachment, identity, comfort, occupation and inclusion (see Figure 5.1). As dementia progresses a person may rely more on other people to get these core needs met.

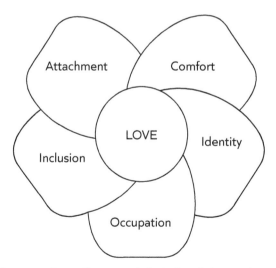

Figure 5.1: Kitwood's core psychological needs (Kitwood 1997)

Kitwood's model advocates that appropriate use of communication and behaviour can contribute to sustaining the core psychological needs of people with dementia. Person-centred communication is the process of applying these principles. What we say and how we say it can make a positive or negative difference to the wellbeing of the person with dementia.

An example of how ill-considered communication can impact on a person's core psychological needs is illustrated in the case of Anira. The needs of attachment and comfort are negated in the brief inter-action between Anira and the care worker. The care worker did not acknowledge Anira's distress through not engaging with her reality and emotions. Anira was not listened to or given the time needed to attempt to explain her situation when she was already frustrated by word-finding difficulties. The care worker then went on to 'infantilize' Anira (treating her as if she were a child) by placing her arm on her and instructing her to 'come with me'. This exacerbated Anira's distress which could have been ameliorated with a different approach.

For example, using the approach of 'validation' (accepting the truth of a person's reality and feelings and communicating that acceptance) the care worker might have responded to Anira with something like 'You are looking for Rohan, you must feel worried without him here?' This would have had the effect of letting Anira know that her distress and the reasons for it were recognized and understood, possibly resulting in a feeling of relief, rather than further frustration, and may have allowed the care worker to offer reassurance and distraction to help Anira in that moment.

To effectively apply person-centred communication, an under-standing of the history and wider context of a person's life beyond that of their dementia is also necessary, allowing for the develop-ment of empathy, and the building of a therapeutic relationship. In the case of Anira, knowing that she is often looking for Rohan, and that she needs time to communicate due to her word-finding diffi-culties, makes approaching communication with her easier. Correct use of body language is important because, if used insensitively, it can negatively affect attempts at person-centred communication. If the care worker had demonstrated active listening and an open posture (i.e., no crossed arms and turned towards the person), that alone may have provided some reassurance to Anira and put her at ease, making the interaction that followed easier for them both. Modern-day time pressures often demand multi-tasking and time-saving strategies; for example, rushing someone to the dining hall or typing information into a computer during a consultation. This body language alone can contribute to feelings of invalidation, anxiety and self-doubt and is likely to cost time in the long run, if communication is ineffective.

STRATEGIES FOR SUPPORTING COMMUNICATION WHEN APHASIA IS PRESENT

Aphasia is a feature of all types of dementia. Language can be affected early on in some types of dementia, whereas many people develop aphasia as the disease advances. Anira demonstrates expressive aphasia when searching for words that she cannot express. Receptive aphasia refers to difficulties understanding and processing language. People with aphasia may become frustrated because they cannot express words denoting objects (anomia), generate sentences with relevant words (non-fluent aphasia), or they produce sentences that make no sense (fluent aphasia). Some people with aphasia have reduced insight into their difficulties creating more frustration for those caring for them.

For those with insight into their aphasia, language difficulties may affect self-esteem because social interactions and relationships are seen to define us as human beings. Sometimes distressed behaviours are borne out of frustration due to restrictions on verbal expression. This expression of need is often classed as being seen to be due to 'the dementia', instantly closing avenues to implement interventions that enhance communication, as seen in the dialogue with Anira. Active listening is paramount and serves a dual purpose, listening fully to the person to understand both their needs and perspective which serves to validate them and their reality without judgement (Alsawy et al. 2020). Make sure you allow enough time for interactions, to allow for the person's delayed processing and information retrieval difficulties. This takes pressure from the practitioner and so allows for a positive intervention. It is possible in many cases to infer missed words or understand the concept of a poorly generated sentence by listening to tone, pitch and emotion. Asking questions for clarification shows empathy and empowers the person with dementia, as opposed to finishing their sentences and making assumptions.

A common mistake made by professionals is in taking what is said at face value. A classic example is asking a person with dementia if they are in pain. The person might respond with 'no' when they mean 'yes'. It is important for healthcare professionals to consistently assess body language, and discuss with family and relevant others so that verbal information can be corroborated. Body language observation is vital when communicating with people with dementia to identify discomfort or frustration. Perseveration is a neurological symptom that concerns repetition of certain behaviours, sounds or words. This can be confusing because perseveration might be mistaken for an expression of discomfort, for example repeatedly saying 'no' or shouting a specific phrase. Positive, respectful and empowering conversations can allow for greater empathy and communication that encourages validation and acceptance for the person with dementia and a more meaningful intervention.

STRATEGIES FOR SUPPORTING COMMUNICATION WHEN A PERSON IS NON-VERBAL

For some people with dementia, as the disease advances, the ability to communicate verbally may be completely lost. This can also happen earlier in the disease for people with certain types of dementia, for example in primary progressive aphasia. When verbal communication is challenged in this way the person might only be able to make sounds and broken words, or they may rely entirely on gestures and body language to communicate. It is important to note that a person who is non-verbal may also have problems with comprehension, and information may need to be gained from family carers or professionals who know the person well.

Communicating with someone who is non-verbal can feel challenging, and so it is important to have a 'toolkit' of approaches you can use to enhance communication in these circumstances. It can be beneficial to take on an investigative role by asking relevant questions to family or professional carers to understand what might be happening for the person with dementia. Again, a thorough history and body language observations are informative foundations on which to generate hypotheses or a rationale for a behaviour. If a person is refusing to eat, questions to consider might be: When was the last dental check? Is the person being offered their preferred diet and food choices? Does evidence suggest a change in taste? (as can be experienced in some people with dementia). Is the mealtime environment noisy or confusing? Does stress influence their mealtime experience? Box 5.2 provides some further useful tips for communicating when someone has lost the ability to communicate verbally.

Box 5.2: Tips for communication when someone is non-verbal

→ When talking directly with the person with dementia, it is important to remain calm and speak softly and kindly.

→ Use short sentences, speak slowly and at a volume the person is likely to hear. Ultimately, remember that everyone is different in how they communicate.

→ Give the person time – longer than you might usually to wait for a response.

→ Consider the environment and keep distractions to a minimum (e.g., turning off the television).

→ Various methods are available to support the person to communicate needs – consider things like communication cards or using yes/no questions if the person can use gestures like shaking the head to communicate.

→ Behaviour is often a means of communication when a person is non-verbal; be prepared to read any unusual or distress behaviours and interpret what they might mean.

→ Gentle touch can be a powerful intervention to reassure and facilitate a safe environment.

→ Positioning is also important; when busy, it can be tempting to stay standing when the person is sitting. Interacting at eye level will yield a better communicative response and it is less intimidating than being looked down at from a height.

(Adapted from Pepper and Harrison Dening 2023)

STRATEGIES FOR COMMUNICATION WHEN THERE ARE FALSE BELIEFS, DELUSIONS OR HALLUCINATIONS

False beliefs, delusions and hallucinations are common and sometimes distressing symptoms of dementia as demonstrated in the case of Ahmed. Auditory, visual and sensory feedback can all be distorted by dementia, which can impact on a person's perception of their environment. On some level, there may be an awareness that their perception is faulty so when challenged, delusions might solidify, resulting in distressed behaviours. As we see with Ahmed, his beliefs feel incredibly real to him. In other cases, symptoms might be more flexible, and the individual open to having their beliefs gently challenged. It is important to continually assess the person's presentation and mood to predict how to proceed with any discussion about their beliefs. It can be helpful to focus on and explore their presenting emotions rather than the beliefs themselves, bearing in mind that the person's level of understanding and comprehension is restricted.

In the example of Ahmed, an understanding of his life story might reveal a historical basis for the symptoms he is experiencing, thus making it easier for the district nurses to both understand and accept Ahmed's reality. This might enable them to reassure him and help in their understanding of any historical triggers and emotions that might be influencing current symptoms. As sensory perception becomes distorted, it is important to ensure that people have access to regular tests for vision and hearing and appropriate aids if required. If an environment is overwhelming and overcluttered or inappropriately lit, it may have an impact on symptoms and processing abilities as the ability to focus attention in dementia is faulty, and the person may be easily distracted.

It is worth bearing in mind that even if a communication strategy is effective on one occasion, it does not follow that it will be effective on another occasion. Many variables, including presenting symptoms, affective state, physiological differences and interpersonal relations, may influence how well the person responds to an intervention. Communication can be unpredictable with people who have dementia and who experience these complex symptoms, but it is important to persevere and be guided by clinical judgement.

COMMUNICATING WITH FAMILY CARERS

Caring for someone with dementia can have a huge impact on a person's emotional and physical wellbeing, as well as having a significant financial impact, for example if they have had to give up work to care. In addition, feelings of guilt may lead to carers neglecting their own needs, placing them at risk of burnout and ill health. At times, family carers might come across as defensive or with high expressed emotion. These emotions are often amplified by the barriers they face when trying to access health and social care services, sometimes causing them to withdraw from services and support, leaving them susceptible to increased risks. All these factors need to be considered when you are approaching any communication with a family member.

We can see some of these factors reflected in the case of Anna and Mary. Although Anna appears to have been given the information that Mary is approaching end of life, this information may not have been given in a way that Anna has been able to fully understand and take in, or the emotional impact of that communication may have been too great, and Anna is in denial. When communicating with family carers, particularly when giving difficult information, it is important to consider the emotional weight of that communication, to check understanding and to offer emotional support as part of the information giving.

Dementia is a progressive terminal disease that requires health and social care professionals to impart difficult information at various times over the trajectory of the condition. For example, at the point of diagnosis, advising the person to stop driving (see Chapter 13), suggesting domiciliary care or admission to care home and end-of-life discussions. Imparting such information in an insensitive or rushed manner may exacerbate complex emotions. Information that may seem benign, such as suggesting the uptake of domiciliary care, could elicit complex emotions for the person and their carer, who may now have to consider letting strangers into their home, and for the carer relinquishing some of their previous caring role. Difficult information conveyed on any level requires the health and social care professional to be vigilant to unspoken responses, remain compassionate and empathic, to gauge body language, ask questions and be aware that there may be questions people are too overwhelmed to consider in that moment. Therefore, providing written information to refer to, encouraging people to take notes and giving contact details for someone they can go to with questions are all important considerations.

Where there are high levels of expressed emotion in communication with family carers, a respectful and patient approach should be used, utilizing skills of active listening, empathy and compassion. Often, simply listening to the challenges family carers experience may make a powerful difference because they often feel isolated in their role. The high level of stress and isolation may mean that some family carers just need to vent their worries and concerns. Facilitating space to discuss their worries is a valuable intervention. Most families have a strong knowledge of the person with dementia; therefore, it is important that families are included in the caring process, in balance with respect, autonomy and independence for the person with dementia.

SUPPORTING COMMUNICATION BETWEEN THE PERSON WITH DEMENTIA AND THE FAMILY CARER

When working with a family with dementia, there may also be the opportunity to support communication between the person with dementia and their family carer. Whilst we know that caring for someone living with dementia can have a substantial negative impact on both physical and mental health, we also know that with the right support caring can be a rewarding experience. Research has shown that family carers of those with dementia can experience communication challenges related to the dementia, a summary of which can be seen in Table 5.1.

Table 5.1: Communication challenges for family carers (adapted from Morris et al. 2020)

Understanding change	Difficulty understanding and coming to terms with changes, and lack of a shared understanding of those changes if the person with dementia does not have insight.
Language	Language changes (e.g., repetitive conversation) can be a source of frustration.
Changes in empathy	Where the person with dementia is struggling to infer the carer's mental state based on non-verbal cues there can be a feeling that the carer is not being recognized for all they are doing.
Role changes and dependence	This can lead to changes in pre-existing communication patterns, which can be difficult to navigate.
Anticipatory grief	Carers may also be experiencing a grief reaction, with obvious complications for communication with a person whom they are also grieving the loss of.
Practical pressures	Practical pressures, fatigue and social isolation can increase stress, making communication more tense. It can also be difficult to find time to access support and learn coping strategies.
Attachment	Being in an 'attachment relationship' (e.g., spouses or a parent/child relationship) can make it difficult to maintain the emotional distance needed to communicate calmly and effectively.

It is important to consider family carers in the context of the above challenges that they might be facing and know where to refer them for support if challenges are identified. Admiral Nurses are specialist dementia nurses who support the whole family. Where there is no local Admiral Nurse available support may be sought through secondary mental health services or other voluntary sector services. There is also a national Admiral Nurse Dementia Helpline and virtual clinics which can offer support and advice (see Resources section).

CONCLUSION

People with dementia will experience communication problems, with the ability to express and receive verbal communication becoming more impaired over time. As health and social care professionals, we need to understand the individual's circumstances, try to decipher why someone is behaving in a certain way and determine if there is a historical connection. It is paramount that the family are involved and communicated with throughout so long as this is balanced with the autonomy, wishes and respect for the person with dementia. This can be difficult for professionals, when faced with work demands, shortages of staff, lack of resources, all of which impinge on our ability to spend the time we would like with the people in our care. Despite this, we can employ certain actions and communication approaches that will facilitate an environment of safety, compassion and validation for the person with dementia and their family carers.

SOURCES OF SUPPORT

If you have any questions about helping a person with any aspect of dementia, call our free Helpline on 0800 888 6678 or email at helpline@dementiauk.org
If you would prefer a pre-booked appointment by phone or video, call via the Dementia UK website: www.dementiauk.org

RESOURCES

Dementia UK. **Tips for communicating with a person with dementia.** www.dementiauk.org/wp-content/uploads/2023/07/dementia-uk-communication-tips.pdf
Dementia UK. **False beliefs and delusions in dementia.** www.dementiauk.org/wp-content/uploads/dementia-uk-false-beliefs-delusions.pdf
SCIE. **Behaviour in dementia as a form of communication.** www.scie.org.uk/dementia/after-diagnosis/communication/behaviour.asp

REFERENCES

Alsawy, S., Tai, S., McEvoy, P. & Mansell, W. (2020) It's nice to think somebody's listening to me instead of saying 'oh shut up': People with dementia reflect on what makes communication good and meaningful. *Journal of Psychiatric and Mental Health Nursing.* 27(2): 151–161.
Kitwood, T. (1997) The experience of dementia. *Aging & Mental Health.* 1(1): 13–22.
Morris, L., Mansell, W., Williamson, T., Wray, A. & McEvoy, P. (2020) Communication Empowerment Framework: An integrative framework to support effective communication and interaction between carers and people living with Dementia. *Dementia.* 19(6): 1739–1757. doi:10.1177/1471301218805329
Pepper, A. & Dening, K.H. (2023) Person-centred communication with people with dementia. *Nursing Older People.* https://doi.org/10.7748/nop. 2023.e1430

CHAPTER 6

Understanding behaviours in care homes

INTRODUCTION

Some people with dementia may get agitated and distressed but are unable to communicate this verbally and, in these cases, this distress can be presented as a change in behaviour. Families and staff may need specialist help and support to identify the probable cause, in order to devise a person-centred plan to prevent or manage the distress. The example below provided by nurse Sarra Blackman demonstrates some of the difficulties that can be experienced by nurses in caring for people with dementia in a care home. Following this, a specialist dementia nurse (Admiral Nurse) explores how to provide care for people with dementia in a care home setting.

Sarra Blackman, Community Psychiatric Nurse, Older Adult Mental Health Team

Charlie, a resident in a care home, had started to regularly lie on the floor throughout the day. Charlie was not falling; he chose to lie on the floor. This caused concern for the care home staff as this was felt to be a behaviour that was not only difficult to understand but was also placing Charlie and other residents at risk. The care home manager and the team felt that Charlie would injure himself or others, or even that he would become ill and catch a cold by lying on the floor. Similarly, seeing Charlie on the floor caused visitors to question the level of care that residents were receiving. The care home owners were also concerned about how this behaviour was perceived by professionals and tradespeople coming to the home, in addition to family visitors. Attempts to encourage Charlie to lie in bed or sit in a chair were unsuccessful and caused Charlie to become distressed, especially when the team attempted to hoist him from the floor against his will.

The care home team turned to Charlie's GP for help which led to a referral to the Older Adult Community Mental Health Team. Naturally, part of the screening criteria for a referral was that any underlying physical health problems had been considered to rule out any reversible causes for changes in his presentation. Results of all tests came back normal. So, Charlie was not experiencing any physical health change that would explain this change in presentation.

At the time I was working as a Community Psychiatric Nurse with the Older Adult Mental Health Team, and I was allocated the referral to my caseload. On assessment Charlie was not presenting with any state of distress. His communication and understanding were impaired as his degree of cognitive decline was moderate to severe. This meant that direct questioning of Charlie was not possible. I was able to assess for pain but did not elicit the presence of any and reviewed Charlie's daily notes which showed no concerns regarding food and fluid intake, elimination or sleep pattern. I questioned the staff about Charlie's care and their perceptions of his behaviours and they were at a loss to explain the change, but importantly felt the reason he was behaving in this way was because they were failing to care properly for him.

Nikki Rowe, Academy Admiral Nurse

In order to be able to assess and provide best practice support to Charlie, his family and the team who care for him, it would be useful to have some further information about his dementia diagnosis. For example, does Charlie have a formal diagnosis of dementia, and if so, what is the type of dementia and when was he diagnosed? This information can be obtained from the GP surgery if the care home does not have access to his clinical summary. Having this information will support Charlie's assessment by giving a clear indication of his dementia history and where he is in his journey living with dementia. It would also be helpful to know if Charlie has any history of mental health conditions such as anxiety or depression, as his behaviours now may be indicative of the way he is feeling, particularly if he has newly transitioned into the home and is adjusting to his new environment.

During her review, Sarra reviewed Charlie's pain levels and felt this was not the cause of his change in behaviour. It would also be helpful to assess Charlie for any other possible physical causes for his behaviour, such as delirium, infection or constipation. This may be done by taking a simple urinalysis to check for a urinary tract infection, observing for symptoms of a chest infection or constipation.

When supporting a care home team, the Admiral Nurse would try to establish the possible underlying reasons for Charlie's behaviour to be able to advise on how best to prevent or manage what is happening. One assessment approach that could be used is the '**ABC**' tool which helps to identify triggers for the observed behaviour by monitoring environmental and internal factors which occur before the behaviour (**A**ntecedent), the **B**ehaviour observed and the **C**onsequences of the behaviour. Use of an ABC behavioural chart would enable the care team to monitor, document and evidence reasons and triggers (Dobbs et al. 2022). This, in turn, would assist in planning Charlie's care centred around his needs. If triggers were identified by using the ABC chart, it may be possible to identify the cause of Charlie's distress and find preventative measures to reduce the consequences. Ideally the ABC chart should be recorded for a period of at least three weeks to establish the frequency of Charlie's displayed distress and to allow for any patterns to emerge.

It is also important to establish if this is a new behaviour or whether it was occurring before Charlie was admitted to the care home. To establish this, the care staff or Admiral Nurse (if one is available) could speak with Charlie's family and ask their opinion about when he began to act in this way, why he may be doing this and what, if anything, they found would prevent or help reduce the behaviour.

If Charlie's behaviour is new, then thinking about any changes in his life may also help us to understand the reason for his behaviour. Sarra has identified that there had been no physical changes in his presentation, but that it was possible that there had been emotional changes that Charlie was reacting to. Changes such as his family circumstances, environment or even care routine may be distressing to Charlie, particularly as his memory is poor and he is struggling to understand or make sense of these changes; therefore he may be expressing this distress through his behaviour as he may be unable to express it in any other way.

COMMUNICATION WITH THE CARE HOME TEAM AND APPROACHES THEY COULD USE

The care home team should be supported in understanding the importance of demonstrating understanding and patience when Charlie is distressed. They should also be encouraged to explore why Charlie could be presenting in this way, to enhance their understanding and help them to think of ways to prevent or better manage his distress (Rapaport et al. 2018). Part of this will also involve helping the care team to consider and share different ways to prevent the distress, such as establishing if there is a time of day when Charlie is more distressed and implementing strategies before he gets into a distressed state, for example playing relaxing music, taking a walk in the garden, or a cup of tea and a snack. Care staff may be able to offer sensory support such as a hand massage (if appropriate) to offer comforting touch, or they may need to give Charlie space but observe at a safe distance. Different approaches can be tried with Charlie to establish which works best for him and this can then be incorporated into his care plan.

Staff would need support, practical advice and perhaps even role modelling on how to care for Charlie during an episode of distress. This may consist of sitting with Charlie, and offering verbal reassurance and comfort to try to avoid his distress escalating. It is important that the team remain as calm as possible and try not to crowd him, instead taking a relaxed one-person approach, especially if the one person is a staff member that Charlie knows and trusts.

KNOWING A PERSON'S LIFE STORY

The benefits of life story work can be explained to the staff, along with guidance on how this can be structured and applied in Charlie's case. The staff could ask Charlie about his life, interests, employment and family. If he is unable to share this with the staff, then his family could help provide this information to enable the development and construction of his life story. A better understanding of Charlie's life story may be the key to understanding the root cause of his distress or it may aid in finding an intervention that is meaningful to him that can be used to support him during a time of distress. Using information about Charlie's life, such as his childhood, his job, family life and hobbies, will help the staff to understand that Charlie is a whole person who has a past that could shape the present and future (Gridley et al. 2020), but may also have a reassuring effect on Charlie in that he feels safe and comforted that this person seems to know him. An example of using Charlie's life story to support his emotional wellbeing would be if he used to play guitar in a band, then using music from a similar era may help him to feel calm and a sense of relaxation at times of feeling overwhelmed. By taking what they know about Charlie and incorporating this into his care plan it becomes person-centred care.

COMMUNICATION WITH CHARLIE'S FAMILY

Charlie's family are likely to be frightened and confused by his change in behaviour, especially if this is a new distress reaction, and will need support to understand why this may be happening. Offering a face-to-face meeting with Charlie's family could help explain that the care home is making attempts to investigate why these changes are happening. As previously mentioned, the family could also be asked if Charlie had had any similar episodes before, and if so, were there any approaches which worked to prevent or reduce Charlie's distress. The care plan could also be discussed with the family and their involvement with this would be welcomed.

The family could also be asked about Charlie's diagnosis and progression to date to establish their own understanding of his dementia. It is likely that Charlie's family may require ongoing support during this time. Good communication between the care home team, other professionals involved, and Charlie's family is likely to be instrumental in finding what interventions and care approaches work best to reduce his distress, which demonstrates the importance of relationships between care staff, Charlie and his family.

PERSON-CENTRED PLAN

Having a robust care plan which includes aspects of Charlie's life story, his needs and wishes, and also considering the wishes of his family, will put in place all the building blocks needed to enable the care team to meet his needs in a person-centred way that will support a sense of wellbeing for Charlie (Cooney and O'Shea, 2019). When the staff have an understanding about Charlie's life and how this has shaped him, they might be more aware of why he is expressing himself in this way currently. They can then devise ways to meet his needs in a more focused and person-centred way.

CONCLUSION

Focusing on the probable causes of behaviour and planning to prevent or reduce these can lead to a reduction of distress behaviours and a better quality of life for the person with dementia. These identified approaches and interventions can be written into a person-centred care plan for a resident so all staff can implement them. Establishing and managing the causes of distress through planned, psychosocial interventions can also reduce the need for the use of unnecessary antipsychotic medication.

SOURCES OF SUPPORT

If you have any questions about helping a person with any aspect of dementia, call our free Helpline on 0800 888 6678 or email at helpline@dementiauk.org
If you would prefer a pre-booked appointment by phone or video, call via the Dementia UK website: www.dementiauk.org

RESOURCES

Dementia UK. **Creating a life story.** www.dementiauk.org/get-support/living-with-dementia/creating-a-life-story/

Using the ABC approach and making a plan to tackle difficult behaviours in dementia. www.psychologytoday.com/gb/blog/managing-your-memory/202202/use-antecedents-and-consequences-manage-dementia-behaviors

REFERENCES

Cooney, A. & O'Shea, E. (2019) The impact of life story work on person-centred care for people with dementia living in long-stay care settings in Ireland. *Dementia.* 18(7–8): 2731–2746.

Dobbs, D., Zimmerman, P.C., Beeber, A.S. et al. (2022) Staff reports of behavioural expressions of persons with dementia in 250 Assisted Living Communities. *The Gerontologist.* 62(2): 169–180.

Gridley, K., Birks, Y. & Parker, G. (2020) Exploring good practice in life story work with people with dementia: The findings of a qualitative study looking at the multiple views of stakeholders. *Dementia.* 19(2): 182–194.

Rapaport, P., Livingston, G., Hamilton, O. et al. (2018) How do care home staff understand, manage and respond to agitation in people with dementia? A qualitative study. *BMJ Open.* 8(6): e022260. http://dx.doi.org/10.1136/bmjopen-2018-022260

CHAPTER 7

Managing the risk of getting lost or going missing

'FATHER SHOULD NOT BE ALLOWED OUT ALONE'

INTRODUCTION

Due to issues with memory, orientation and communication associated with cognitive decline people living with dementia can experience symptoms that can lead them to get lost, for example if they go out and forget where they were going or become disorientated with their surroundings. It is estimated that more than 40,000 people living with dementia go missing for the first time each year but only a minority go missing frequently (National Police Improvement Agency (2011). The risk of getting lost or going missing is often a cause for concern for people living with dementia, their families, carers and professionals alike. These concerns are not unfounded; whilst the majority of people living with dementia who go missing are found safe and well, it is recognized that some do come to serious harm or suffer injuries that can result in death.

Such serious negative outcomes, although uncommon, can create an environment whereby once any potential or actual risk has been identified, there is a propensity to try and eradicate any perceived risk of harm. This can lead to restrictions being placed upon a person's freedom as those who care for them can sometimes resort to restrictive strategies in an attempt to keep the person physically safe, and this may even result in a premature admission to residential care (Bantry-White and Montgomery 2015). However, such imposed restrictions may not be in the person's best interests and accepting a degree of risk may be needed to promote patient autonomy and well-being (Clarke and Mantle 2016), particularly as walking and exercise have been identified as important factors in living well with dementia (Shalev Greene et al. 2019).

This case study provides an account from a community nurse who supported a family carer when her husband went missing. This is followed by advice from a dementia nurse consultant who discusses some of the key issues relating to risk assessment and safeguarding and the benefits of a proactive approach to risk assessment.

Deiondre Jackson, Community Nurse (pseudonym)

Thomas is a 75-year-old man who was diagnosed with Alzheimer's disease by the local memory assessment service 18 months ago. He was not suitable for cholinesterase inhibitors due to a cardiac problem and was discharged straight back to the care of his GP after diagnosis. Thomas declined any follow-up support from the local dementia support service stating he just wanted to get on with his life.

Thomas lives with his partner Libby in a remote house in a rural village. They have been in a close relationship for the past seven years but have been friends for over 30 years. Thomas' first wife Sara died nine years ago. Libby is 73 years old and is also widowed; her husband died 12 years ago. Both have two children from previous relationships.

Prior to the move to their current home, they lived in a large city approximately 50 miles away, where many of their family and friends remain. Thomas likes to be outdoors and to go walking to engage with nature which was one of the reasons for the move to a village. However, Libby has restricted mobility as she has chronic obstructive pulmonary disease (COPD) which prevents her from walking very far, hence Thomas often goes out walking alone. Until recently they enjoyed a very active social life as a couple and volunteered at a food bank in a nearby town. Whilst they have tried to continue to participate in social activities and volunteering this has become more difficult as Thomas had to stop driving three months ago. Thomas sometimes gets a lift with friends or neighbours, but Libby tends to stay at home.

I have been supporting Libby for several months to monitor her COPD but also to apply dressings to her ulcerated legs. I started visiting her at home when it became more difficult for her to attend the practice. On a recent visit to their home, I arrived to find Libby in a distressed state. Libby advised me that Thomas had gone out for a walk over three hours earlier and had not returned. Libby had no idea where he might be and was concerned as it was getting very cold outside.

I asked if he might have popped into a neighbour's house. Libby said she had tried everyone she could think of, but no one had seen him. I suggested that Libby call the police to report Thomas missing; although reluctant, she agreed. Libby also alerted Thomas' two sons, Colin and Jack, to the situation. I advised Thomas' GP of the situation and made a safeguarding referral to adult social services with Libby's consent. I had met Thomas on several occasions and had never had cause for concern about his safety prior to this occasion.

Colin and Jack were worried about their father's wellbeing, so travelled home to monitor the situation, planning to stay for a few days to see what could be done to prevent it happening again.

The police found Thomas safe and well a few hours later at a railway station after being alerted by a member of the public. He had been waiting for a train to bring him back from the city where they had previously lived. The police returned Thomas home where Libby and his two sons were waiting. The following day the family were visited by a social worker, and I was also asked to attend. Libby advised that she was doing her best to support Thomas to be as independent as possible and enable him to do the things that he enjoyed whilst he was still able, as per his wishes. The sons felt their father should not be allowed out alone and as Libby was unable to go out for a walk, felt he should only go out if someone was with him. Thomas stated that if he was no longer able to go out for a walk on his own, he might as well end his life, stating that going for a walk and being out in the fresh air helped his mood and made him feel alive and without that he could see little meaning in his life.

The social worker assessed Thomas as having mental capacity to make decisions relating to going out alone as he could under-stand the risks that he could face if he got lost again and was able to articulate a wider set of risks that he felt would be relevant to him should he not be allowed to go out walking.

It was also considered that because Thomas lives with Libby, she could raise the alarm if he did not return when planned. This was good, because if Thomas lived alone, it might be some time before someone realized he was missing. Colin and Jack were anxious about the decision but recognized that their father had the right to make this decision and, despite living with dementia, was able to make choices which they might not agree with. It also prompted them to offer more practical support to their father and Libby and commit to visiting more regularly to take them both out.

The social worker put some risk reduction strategies in place, such as arranging an assistive technology referral to consider a tracking device for Thomas to wear when he goes out. Thomas was agreeable to this although he jokingly added that 'I will take it off when I visit the girlfriend.' The police have asked Libby and Thomas to fill in a 'Herbert Protocol' which I had not heard of before, which is a document that holds key information about Thomas to help the police search for him if he ever goes missing again. It has been agreed that the risk will be monitored and regularly reviewed as things are likely to change as time goes by. I am relieved that this is the outcome, but I have spent a lot of time reflecting on whether I missed something and could have prevented this event from happening and what I would do differently if faced with a similar situation again.

(Pseudonyms have been used to ensure anonymity of the nurse and people with dementia and their family.)

Dr Zena Aldridge, Independent Dementia Nurse Consultant (formerly Admiral Nurse Research Fellow)

Risk assessment and risk management are vital in supporting people living with dementia, their families and carers both in terms of identifying behaviours that pose a risk to the person with dementia, but also any risks posed to others. However, health and social care professionals are likely to focus on risks associated within the scope of their role, for example adopting a mental health, physical health or social care perspective to risk.

Furthermore, the concept of risk is subjective and what is seen to constitute a risk can be influenced by the knowledge and skill set of the professional as well as the context of a given situation, such as where the person with dementia is at any given point in time, and what, if any, support they are receiving. The perception of risk may also be influenced by a person's beliefs, values and unique life history (Department of Health (DH) 2010; Kitwood 1995; Sandberg et al. 2017). Clarke and colleagues (2011: 11) described risk in the context of dementia care as having 'multiple meanings for multiple people in multiple situations'.

In Thomas' case, the contextual factors are likely to have influenced decision-making; for example, he did not live alone. Living with Libby was a protective factor in reducing some of the risk should he go missing or get lost in the future, as she could raise the alarm at the earliest opportunity. Thomas had the mental capacity to weigh up the risks and make an informed decision about how to prospectively manage future risk. Thomas articulated clearly that preventing him from going out for a walk would create risks in other areas, so preventing him from going out independently may reduce the risk of him getting lost, but the inability to make choices and retain his autonomy would have a detrimental impact on his social, emotional and psychological wellbeing and his mental health.

POSITIVE RISK TAKING

To inform a person-centred approach to risk management it is important to consider the underpinning principles of positive risk taking and risk enablement. Risk enablement has four main aims (Clarke and Mantle 2016; Clarke et al. 2011):

- To enable people to manage uncertainty rather than create certainty and to avoid unnecessary dependence and risk avoidance.

- To effectively advocate for the views of the person with dementia and involve them in decisions about risk taking or risk avoidance.

- To ensure that the risk assessment includes psychosocial and emotional wellbeing as well as physical safety.

- To ensure that there is effective communication within and between services.

This approach aims to protect the identity, agency, and purpose of a person's life by alleviating the risk of what Clarke and colleagues (2011) describe as the 'silent harms' caused when risk-aversive approaches lead to a person with dementia feeling unfulfilled, bored, frustrated and lacking the ability to be autonomous. It is of course recognized that the outcome will not always be the same as there is a need to contextualize the risk so that vulnerable people with dementia are supported but also protected.

Contextual determinants will be different for each person and can change over time which is why it is critical that risk assessment is seen as an ongoing process and not a one-off 'tick box' exercise. It is important to recognize that identifying a risk does not necessarily make you responsible for assessing and managing that risk, particularly if it is out of your normal sphere of practice. What is important is that health and social care professionals recognize their roles and responsibilities in escalating any concerns about risk through appropriate referral routes. Where necessary this may require the sharing of information to inform risk assessments, management plans and aid shared collaborative decision-making to safeguard those in your care, as is illustrated in the case study of Thomas.

SAFEGUARDING

When considering risk in the context of dementia care, it is important to make sure any safeguarding concerns are addressed. The six principles of safeguarding – accountability, prevention, protection, partnership, proportionality, empowerment – are embedded within the Care Act (2014) (see Table 7.1). Following these principles also supports person-centred decision making as they align with the four key issues relating to risk enablement as discussed earlier, particularly when the risk is subjective and there are no objective measures to assess the level of risk to an individual.

Table 7.1: The six principles of Safeguarding (adapted
from Social Care Institute for Excellence 2023)

Empowerment	People should be supported and encouraged to make their own decisions and professionals should seek informed consent.
Prevention	It is better to be proactive rather than wait for harm to occur.
Proportionality	The least restrictive and intrusive response to risk should be adopted.
Protection	There must be support and representation for those in greatest need to protect them from harm.
Partnership	Services should work collaboratively to find local solutions. Communities have a part to play in preventing, detecting and reporting neglect and abuse.
Accountability	There is a need for accountability and transparency in safeguarding practice.

In the case of Thomas, the level of risk was subjective, however Deiondre recognized her **accountability** within the situation as a registered nurse who had come across a situation where a potentially vulnerable adult could be at risk of significant harm and who may need **protection**. Consequently, her response was **proportionate** to the possible risks, and by making a safeguarding referral, contacting the GP and encouraging Libby to report Thomas missing to the police, she took a **partnership** approach in trying to respond to this situation. Because of Deiondre's actions, the police and social worker were able to respond to the concerns in a timely manner and employ **preventive** and **proportionate** strategies that adopted a risk enablement approach and protected Thomas' right to autonomy. Thomas was therefore **empowered** and supported in the decision-making process and in the adoption of strategies which could reduce the risk of him going missing in the future.

MENTAL CAPACITY ACT

It is important that any risk assessments or safeguarding decisions are considered within the context of a person's unique history, and it should not be assumed that a bad decision about risk behaviours is inevitable when there is a diagnosis of dementia, and the principles of the Mental Capacity Act (MCA) (DH 2005) should be applied to inform practice.

The MCA (DH 2005) offers an objective legal framework for assessing a person's understanding and processing of the relevant information and their ability to retain it long enough for them to be able to make a decision and subsequently communicate a choice. The MCA (DH 2005) is clear that capacity is time and decision specific and that capacity can fluctuate so there may be a need to revisit decisions as a person's capacity changes. If a person is deemed to lack the mental capacity to make decisions, there is a requirement to make decisions on their behalf and in their best interests by adopting the least restrictive options to meet a person's needs. When formulating a best interest decision you must consider the person's wishes and preferences if they are known, what the person may have decided for themselves when they were still able to do so, the different options available, the likely risks of each option including the consideration of any negative risks to the person, how restrictive each option is and how it could impact upon the person's freedom (National institute for Health and Care Excellence (NICE) 2018).

RISK PREVENTION

The best way to manage risk is to take a preventative and proactive approach; it is important that health and social care professionals and families affected by dementia are made aware of any potential risks. An increased awareness can encourage earlier conversations about what the person with dementia's preferences might be and to discuss possible risk management strategies to reduce the risk of, as in this case, going missing. This means improving opportunities for the person with dementia to be involved in decision making and protecting their right to autonomy for as long as possible. The next two sections will introduce two examples of potential possible risk reduction strategies relating to going missing or getting lost.

The Herbert Protocol

The Herbert Protocol was developed in 2011 by Norfolk Police as an initiative to reduce the risk of harm to vulnerable people who may go missing from a care home, but has since been recognized as a valuable tool to support the police search for anyone with dementia who may go missing. It is called the Herbert Protocol after George Herbert, a Second World War veteran who was living with dementia. George died after going missing whilst trying to walk to his childhood home. The Herbert Protocol is now a nationwide scheme which has been adopted by police forces across the country. The Herbert Protocol is a risk reduction tool that consists of a form which contains vital information about the person at risk which can be passed to the police in the event that they go missing. The protocol contains information such as: a physical description, a recent photograph, information about their health, their ability to access transport, their usual routines and places where they might go.

Proactively completing the form ensures key information is readily available which can enable the police to look in the most likely places to find the person as quickly as possible in the event that they go missing. Making a missing person report to the police can be a stressful experience so it is much easier for all if the police have the information to hand in the event of a vulnerable person going missing. The form can be completed when a person is calm and relaxed and hence less likely to omit critical information that could support the police to find the person quickly and safely. Following its introduction, the Herbert Protocol has been used many times to trace missing people with dementia who have then been safely returned home. It is a good example of how emergency and care services can work collaboratively to try and keep people with dementia safe.

Assistive technology

The use of assistive technology (AT) can offer practical solutions to people with dementia, their families and carers in relation to safe walking. AT includes electronic tracking devices (ETDs) which can take on multiple guises, such as smartwatches, mobile phones or fobs, and are increasingly used by carers to offer reassurance should a person with dementia leave the house. However, the use of AT is not without ethical concerns, such as how to balance autonomy and safety, especially when using ETDs. Consequently, the decision to use an ETD should be part of wider discussion and include the principles of safeguarding, risk enablement and the Mental Capacity Act

(DH 2005). The 'gold standard' would be to ensure that people with dementia have conversations about possible risks and ETD solutions at the earliest opportunity following a diagnosis, at a time when they are more likely to be able communicate their wishes and preferences and make an informed decision about the role of ETD in their future care. It must also be considered that the use of ETD may not be suitable for all people with dementia as they may be unable to integrate the use of the device into their routines or there may be issues with GPS coverage in certain remote areas.

There are many AT devices that can support people with dementia to maintain or improve their ability to independently conduct their activities of daily living and reduce risk; you may wish to contact your local authority for more information or to find out how to access an AT assessment to seek appropriate information and guidance.

CONCLUSION

A proactive approach to assessing and managing risk is essential in supporting people living with dementia to retain autonomy and maintain independence for as long as possible. This can be achieved through early identification of any risks and implementation of risk reduction strategies. A thorough risk assessment should consider the person's needs, looking beyond their dementia diagnosis and paying attention to their physical health, psychological and emotional well-being, and the social context of any perceived risk. Whilst there is a need to protect people living with dementia from risks associated with abuse and exploitation from others, it is vital that health and social care professionals do not take a risk-averse approach that impacts negatively on an individual's health and wellbeing. It is important that health and social care professionals are aware of their varying levels of responsibility when it comes to decision making and where necessary seek support and adopt a more collaborative approach to managing risk.

SOURCES OF SUPPORT

If you have any questions about helping a person with any aspect of dementia, call our free Helpline on 0800 888 6678 or email at helpline@dementiauk.org

If you would prefer a pre-booked appointment by phone or video, call via the Dementia UK website: www.dementiauk.org

RESOURCES

Dementia UK. Living aids and assistive technology for a person with dementia. www.dementiauk.org/get-support/living-with-dementia/living-aids-and-assistive-technology

Safe and Found Online. Safeguarding people living with dementia. https://safeandfoundonline.co.uk

Herbert Protocol Form example. www.met.police.uk/SysSiteAssets/media/downloads/central/advice/herbert-protocol/herbert-protocol-form.pdf

Age UK. Safeguarding older people from abuse and neglect. www.ageuk.org.uk/globalassets/age-uk/documents/factsheets/fs78_safeguarding_older_people_from_abuse_fcs.pdf

'Nothing ventured, nothing gained': Risk guidance for people with dementia (DH). https://assets.publishing.service.gov.uk/government/uploads/system/uploads/attachment_data/file/215960/dh_121493.pdf

Enablement in dementia: Practice Tool (2016). www.researchinpractice.org.uk/adults/publications/2016/february/enablement-in-dementia-practice-tool-2016/

REFERENCES

Bantry-White, E. & Montgomery, P. (2015) Dementia, walking outdoors and getting lost: Incidence, risk factors and consequences from dementia-related police missing-person reports. *Aging & Mental Health*. 19(3): 224–230.

The Care Act (2014) www.legislation.gov.uk/ukpga/2014/23/contents/enacted

Clarke, C.L. & Mantle, R. (2016) Using risk management to promote person-centred dementia care. *Nursing Standard*. 30(28): 41–46.

Clarke, C.L., Wilkinson, H., Keady, J. et al. (2011) *Risk assessment and management for living well with dementia*. London: Jessica Kingsley Publishers.

DH (2010) *Nothing ventured, nothing gained: Risk guidance for people with dementia*. London: Department of Health.

Kitwood, T. (1995) Cultures of care: Tradition and change. In: T. Kitwood & S. Benson (Eds.), *The new culture of dementia care*. London: Hawker Publications.

Mental Capacity Act (2005) www.legislation.gov.uk/ukpga/2005/9/introduction

National Police Improvement Agency (2011) *Alzheimer's safe return project*. London: College of Policing.

NICE (2018) *Overview: Decision-making and mental capacity*. www.nice.org.uk/guidance/qs194

Sandberg, L., Rosenberg, L., Sandman P.O. et al. (2017) Risks in situations that are experienced as unfamiliar and confusing – the perspective of persons with dementia. *Dementia*. 16(4): 471–485.

Shalev Greene, K., Clarke, C.L., Pakes, F. et al. (2019) People with dementia who go missing: A qualitative study of family caregivers decision to report incidents to the police. *Policing*. 13(2): 241–253.

Social Care Institute for Excellence (2023) *What are the six principles of safeguarding?* www.scie.org.uk/safeguarding/adults/introduction/six-principles

CHAPTER 8

Understanding behaviours in the hospice

INTRODUCTION

People with dementia are to be found and cared for in many health and social care settings depending on their needs, with hospices being one such care setting. Hospice care aims to improve quality of life and wellbeing for people who have a life-limiting illness or a long-term condition that cannot be cured. Dementia is a life-limiting illness but has struggled to be accorded the same degree of service provision from within the palliative care domain as for other life-limiting illnesses. However, whilst we acknowledge dementia is a life-limiting condition, many people with this diagnosis will experience other co-morbid conditions, such as cancer, that are also life-limiting. Hospice UK rose to the challenge of giving dementia parity with other terminal conditions with their report 'Hospice enabled dementia care' (2015), and proposed hospices build skills and relationships so they can offer care to people with dementia at the end of life.

However, some hospices still struggle to understand and manage some of the behaviours that people with dementia can present with.

The case study below provides an example of how Jenny, a hospice palliative care nurse at the time, faced challenges in providing inpatient hospice care to a person with dementia with complex symptoms of a co-morbid condition. Following this, a specialist dementia nurse (Admiral Nurse) writes about what hospice care professionals can consider when providing care for people who have dementia, whether as the main diagnosis or when co-morbid with another life-limiting condition, such as cancer. The Admiral Nurse will discuss the various issues in the context of the case study of Elaine.

Jenny Butler, Academic Lecturer in Adult Nursing, Bournemouth University (formerly Ward Manager of Oakhaven Hospice)

When I first began to work in the hospice, a primary diagnosis of dementia rarely fitted the criteria for our services, which was standard practice in many hospices. However, we started to receive more referrals for patients with dementia, especially if there was a complex patient or carer need identified.

Hospices are often places of peace and tranquillity. Bedrooms often have direct access to a garden. This can be problematic when trying to observe confused patients at risk of wandering or falling. Of all the bedrooms, only two can be observed from the nurse's station and, if possible, are kept for those requiring greater attention. We have devices to alert staff when patients get up, however sometimes our staffing ratio (especially at night or when very busy) makes it difficult to both observe and respond when a patient does try to walk unaided. Admitting patients who have dementia causes anxiety for staff, especially during busy times when they are unable to see if a patient wanders. There have been times when confused patients have walked into the kitchens, other patient's rooms and even outside of the hospice. Some of the hospice's 'strengths', such as individual private rooms and access to gardens, can also be a 'weakness' when caring for patients who wander internally or externally.

Elaine was in her early 60s and had been diagnosed with motor neurone disease and early onset dementia. Prior to her diagnoses, Elaine was very independent, but as her symptoms worsened she needed more assistance with her activities of daily living; however, Elaine struggled to accept help. Elaine developed swallowing difficulties, but it was agreed that enteral feeding was not in her best interests, the advice being she should eat a soft diet. She found this hard to understand and regularly tried to eat solid foods. After a couple of choking episodes, it was decided to admit her to the hospice inpatient unit for a review of symptoms and to plan for her future care needs.

Elaine did not want to stay at the hospice, so we had to apply for a DoLS (Deprivation of Liberty Safeguards). Soon after admission she would not allow staff to unpack her bags and asked to go home.

Her carer was exhausted and so we could not ask her to stay to help Elaine settle in for the first night (something we have previously done with cognitively impaired patients). Elaine was physically quite able and mobilized unaided and didn't seem to need much rest time so spent most of her time walking about her room, in the corridors and outside. Her first night was difficult as she did not sleep at all and was distressed at the unfamiliar surroundings, so became increasingly tired and agitated. She held her bags close, feeling unsafe and suspicious of anyone who was nearby. Staff tried different approaches to reassure her but she was very focused on 'getting out' and away from us. The night staff spent all night offering distractions in her room (conversations, music, TV), which helped for short periods. However, during the day, when the ward was busier, it was more difficult to dedicate someone to her care. Some hospice patients and their families require staff to be present for long periods of time to provide care, manage symptoms or for psychological support, but not to the degree that Elaine required. Being able to have the time for those who need it is one of the many reasons staff are attracted to work in a hospice environment, but it does make it hard when it doesn't feel like they can understand or meet a patient's needs, such as with Elaine.

After a few days Elaine learnt how to unlock her bedroom door that led to the garden. To exit a bedroom into the garden requires only a turn of the internal lock rather than a key to allow patients and their families to move freely in their own space. Luckily, Elaine was spotted outside, but for the first time since her admission could not be persuaded to return to the ward. She kept walking and ended up in the car park, trying to open car doors saying she was going to drive off. Other staff came out and tried to encourage her to return to the ward, but Elaine was cross, tried to hit a nurse and swore at visitors close by. This resulted in Elaine having 24-hour, one-to-one care to maintain her safety. Whilst this was the safest option for Elaine, it presented staffing resource implications.

Caroline Scates, Deputy Director for Admiral Nurse Development (formerly a Hospice Nurse)

Dementia is the leading cause of death in the UK, yet is often not recognized as a life-limiting illness and, as Jenny describes, hospices have only recently begun to extend their service offer to people with dementia. Palliative care aims to provide an improved quality of life for people with life-limiting illnesses using early assessment and identification of challenges around physical, psychological and spiritual support to improve families' experience towards the end of life, and is therefore an integral part of dementia care.

The hospice environment, as Jenny highlights, offers a calming and less clinical space than that provided in an acute care setting, with gardens, private rooms and a more 'homely' atmosphere. People with complex palliative care needs often require more time, and so hospices generally have higher staffing levels, supplemented by volunteers. For people experiencing cognitive impairment, distress or disorientation, one could see how hospices could offer the perfect space to receive much-needed clinical assessment of complex symptoms.

The importance of knowing a person's history in offering person-centred care in dementia is well understood (Kitwood 1997), though it is not clear from the case study how well the team knew Elaine prior to her admission. Often people are admitted to a hospice in a crisis situation, but ideally getting to know Elaine and her family and what was important to them may have prepared her more for admission. Hearing of how Elaine 'didn't want to stay' and kept her 'bags close, feeling unsafe and suspicious' speaks of someone who was distressed and frightened, with unmet needs. If access to a day service was previously available, Elaine may have been more familiar with her surroundings, helping with her fear of being somewhere unknown, and perhaps some familiar faces to welcome her through the door.

If the admission was planned, Elaine could have taken some photos and familiar objects from home which may have helped her settle, and if Elaine had a 'Life Story' or 'This Is Me' document (see Resources section), staff may have found engaging and communicating with Elaine a little easier. It is interesting that conversations and music helped Elaine settle for short periods over the night shift – taking a more person-centred approach and knowing more about Elaine and the types of music she enjoys may have helped further (McDermott et al. 2014). Sustaining musical and interpersonal connectedness helps support and value who the person is and maintain the quality of their life, and involving family members in developing a personal playlist for Elaine could support this (see Resources section). Also, family members can play a huge part in supporting staff to know and understand a person with dementia better, so perhaps a discussion with Elaine's family about whether being in a shared bay with other people rather than in a room on her own might have lessened her distress and fear could have been helpful.

Jenny mentions how staff felt anxious when people with dementia 'wander', and understandably such anxiety in staff members often comes from a need to manage risk and keep people safe. However, in dementia care, wandering is a term best avoided as it implies that the person is wandering aimlessly without purpose which is often not the case. There will usually be a reason why someone is walking around, and in Elaine's case it is likely she was seeking an exit, looking for a way to get home as she was frightened, and her surroundings were unfamiliar. Jenny goes on to describe a related instance where Elaine was distressed after walking into the hospice car park and started to act in an agitated way.

This incident resulted in staff caring for Elaine by providing one-to-one supervision to keep her safe. One-to-one care and observations are often implemented after a risk-related event has occurred; however, if such an intervention was instigated proactively, such as in spending one-to-one time to get to know Elaine and working on some strategies to share with staff in her care plan, the incident may have been avoided. Distressed behaviours as described in the case study scenario might have been avoided once Elaine became more familiar with staff members and felt safer in her surroundings. However, it sounds like Elaine was distressed from the beginning of her stay as a Deprivation of Liberty Safeguards (DoLS), was applied for, so her unmet needs were evident from the start. The DoLS procedure is prescribed in law when it is necessary to deprive a person of their liberty, such as a resident or patient who lacks capacity to consent to their care and treatment, in order to keep them safe from harm.

Taking time to understand the unmet needs of a person displaying distressed behaviours requires experience, understanding and a sense of professional curiosity to discover what might help, and thinking about how we communicate effectively is vital (see Table 8.1). Distress can have many different causes, such as fear, pain, anxiety, discomfort, hunger, thirst or temperature, and sometimes a small change can make a huge difference.

Table 8.1: Distress behaviours in dementia – tips for communication (see Resources section)

Presentation	Possible reasons for communication	What to consider
The person is upset or angry and can't explain why.	They could be in pain or feeling unwell, or something could be irritating them about their environment, such as noise, bright light or a strong cooking smell. They may be frightened and confused or feeling alone or abandoned. They may feel you are not listening to them or acknowledging their feelings.	Recognize the person's non-verbal behaviours. Validate their feelings, for example by saying, 'I can see you're angry about something – can I help?' Listen to what they say and do not challenge or dismiss their thoughts and feelings. Check for any physical signs such as cuts, bruises, redness or swelling that could be causing pain. Consider whether they may be in discomfort, for example from arthritis, toothache, a headache or infection. Check the environment to see if the temperature, lighting and noise level are comfortable for them. Think about meaningful distracting activities.
The person talks about needing to go to work, even if they are no longer working.	They may need to feel a sense of purpose – that they are useful and needed. They may have found a sense of identity in their working life that they no longer feel or want to reminisce by telling you about their past occupation.	Listen to the person's life experiences. Encourage them to take part in activities that might help them feel useful and purposeful – for example if they used to work in an office, they could help you sort out paperwork, or if they had a practical profession, they could help with simple DIY. Don't worry if it's not done the way you usually do it.

The person is having difficulty following conversations.	Changes in how people identify and process sounds can cause confusion and make it hard to follow conversations.	Try to ensure only one person speaks at a time. Face the person and speak slowly and clearly – people often use body language and lip reading to help them make sense of conversations. Reduce background noise like the TV or radio. Avoid noisy places, and consider moving the person to a quieter area of the hospice if possible.
The person looks confused and doesn't seem to understand you.	This could be due to a reduced level of understanding, difficulty concentrating or too many distractions. Also consider physical assessment of possible infection causing delirium.	Be reassuring, compassionate and gentle. Remind them who you are and what their relationship is to you; try saying or asking something in a different way, for example using shorter sentences and avoiding open-ended questions. Give the person time to process and respond to your question. If appropriate, use touch. Consider the environment. Consider other possible health issues.

Jenny mentions that having time for people who need it is one of the reasons that staff are attracted to work in a hospice environment, but that it is hard when they feel they can't understand or meet a patient's needs such as in Elaine's case. Having an understanding about how to meet the needs of someone with dementia should be no different to understanding the needs of someone with cancer. However, understanding the causes of the distressed behaviour in people with dementia can be a challenge and sometimes feels like a barrier to hospices being inclusive, as care should ultimately depend on the person's needs and not their diagnosis.

Hospice nurses are incredibly experienced in delivering holistic care and are skilled at managing the distress they often see. Encouraging hospices to increase the amount of education in dementia care for all their staff, or taking a step further and hosting an Admiral Nurse to work alongside them in their hospice, may be a welcome development. An increasing number of Admiral Nurses work alongside hospice and palliative and end-of-life care staff to support families affected by dementia.

Palliative care nurses are often very creative when aiming to relieve burdensome symptoms, and one of the reasons for Elaine's admission was around swallowing difficulties. Both of Elaine's diagnoses, motor neurone disease and dementia, can cause difficulty with swallowing (Ershov 2021), so a referral to the local speech and language therapist for a swallowing assessment could be beneficial. Hospices are usually ideal places to be able to offer a variety of soft foods, so a meeting with the catering team to discuss preferences would be an important step. Hospice catering teams often take great pride in producing high-quality home-cooked food and getting to know the person's dietary likes, dislikes and limitations, so they might be able to help Elaine to find foods that are more palatable and manageable. If Elaine was unable to inform staff of her food preferences, or she did not have a This Is Me document to inform staff of this, then it is important to gain this information from family members early in a person's admission. As part of Elaine's holistic physical assessment, it is essential that her mouth hygiene and teeth are reviewed in case these are impeding her swallowing in some way – often this need in people with dementia can be overlooked (Delwel et al. 2018).

CONCLUSION

To conclude, hospices offer person-centred and holistic care, recognizing the role of family carers, for people facing life-limiting illnesses including dementia. Dementia is a global public health concern with numbers of those being diagnosed rising significantly, so ensuring that families receive the support they need is essential. Palliative care helps families to plan for the future as well as offering effective palliation of symptoms alongside kindness, comfort and care from skilled staff. There are significant strengths that hospice care can offer people with a diagnosis of dementia across the disease trajectory, and with a collaborative and innovative approach to meeting the needs of people with dementia, hospices can invest to develop and support their workforce in ensuring that regardless of diagnosis, people have access to excellent palliative care in their communities.

SOURCES OF SUPPORT

If you have any questions about helping a person with any aspect of dementia, call our free Helpline on 0800 888 6678 or email at helpline@dementiauk.org
If you would prefer a pre-booked appointment by phone or video, call via the Dementia UK website: www.dementiauk.org

RESOURCES

Dementia UK. Creating a life story for a person with dementia. www.dementiauk.org/information-and-support/living-with-dementia/creating-a-life-story
Alzheimer's Society. 'This Is Me'. www.alzheimers.org.uk/get-support/publications-factsheets/this-is-me
Playlist for life. www.playlistforlife.org.uk
Dementia UK. Tips for communicating with a person with dementia. www.dementiauk.org/information-and-support/living-with-dementia/tips-for-communication

REFERENCES

Delwel, S., Binnekade, T.T., Perez, R.S.G.M. et al. (2018) Oral hygiene and oral health in older people with dementia: A comprehensive review with focus on oral soft tissues. *Clinical Oral Investigations.* 22(1): 93–108.

Ershov, V.l. (2021) *Dysphagia associated with neurological disorders: Therapy approaches in neurological disorders.* IntechOpen. http://dx.doi.org/10.5772/intechopen.96165

Hospice UK (2015) *Hospice enabled dementia care: First steps.* www.hospiceuk.org/publications-and-resources/hospice-enabled-dementia-care-first-steps

Kitwood, T. (1997) *Dementia reconsidered: The person comes first.* Buckingham: Open University Press.

McDermott, O., Orrell, M. & Ridder, H.M. (2014) The importance of music for people with dementia: The perspectives of people with dementia, family carers, staff and music therapists. *Aging & Mental Health.* 18(6): 706–716.

CHAPTER 9

Challenges when working with someone with dementia in an Emergency Department

INTRODUCTION

When people with dementia have healthcare needs that necessitate an urgent assessment, diagnosis and treatment they may be taken to an Emergency Department (ED). Meeting the needs of people with dementia in EDs can be very challenging for the staff. EDs are by their nature very noisy, brightly lit and busy environments which can increase the feelings of fear, worry and distress for the person with dementia. This in turn can lead to disorientation, agitation, communication difficulties and in some cases aggression as the person with dementia struggles to understand what is happening. It is important that ED staff are skilled in screening, assessing and managing people with dementia to reduce the distress experienced during their attendance at the ED (Manning 2021).

The case study below provided by nurses Melissa and Alexa provides an example of the difficulties that can be experienced when a person with dementia is taken to an ED. Following this a specialist dementia nurse (Admiral Nurse) explores what to do to recognize, prevent and/or manage distress when a person is taken into an ED.

Melissa O'Reilly and Alexa Durham, Registered General Nurses

There are many challenges that ED staff face in caring for people with dementia who arrive in our department. Not least the ED is busy, noisy and bright and can be overwhelming for people with dementia. This can lead to distress, agitation and frustration for the person with dementia and can lead to difficulties in communication with staff.

Another challenge that staff face is in gaining a baseline and history, which can be especially difficult when the patient is brought in alone without a carer or next of kin. For someone with dementia having someone familiar at such a vulnerable and scary time helps them to cope better with the unfamiliar environment, the health issue they have been brought to the ED to seek treatment for, and to provide valuable information on which to base the assessment and treatment.

As members of staff in the ED we have a commitment to making sure family carers have visiting access when patients have dementia, following the guidelines from John's Campaign (see Resources section) and we believe that the best outcomes are achievable when we work in partnership with the family. However sometimes this is difficult to achieve when no next of kin is in attendance to support the patient with dementia.

The ED environment also presents a safety challenge for a person with dementia. It is so busy and there are patients in every area, including the corridors. It is usual for an ED patient to remain in their cubicle or seat as they await assessment and treatment. However, a patient with dementia may not understand this approach to their care. Managing patients who may go walking around the ED is very difficult as there is a lack of space and many obstacles in the form of equipment, and so there is a high risk of falls for people with dementia. In the ED where we work there is only one dedicated cubicle for patients with dementia and this is often in use.

Safe staffing levels may be another challenge – managing patients with complex needs, such as dementia, can impact on our staff to patient ratios. We often have to seek extra staffing resources and use teams such as the Enhanced Care team to optimize patient care in the department.

We know that the ED is not ideally designed for patients with dementia due to it being a fast-paced and noisy environment. We try to create a calm and soothing environment allowing the patient to feel safe, but the additional challenges of working in such a pressured environment with limited resources can impact on the support we are able to offer to patients with dementia.

Chris O'Connor, Consultant Admiral Nurse, East Surrey Hospital

ENVIRONMENTAL ISSUES

Although dementia can affect people across the age range, it predominantly affects older people who are at a higher risk of living with another co-morbidity, such as cardiac conditions, sensory loss, and other long-term conditions. On average the number of co-morbid conditions of people with dementia aged over 65 is double that of those without dementia (Poblador-Plou et al. 2014). For healthcare staff in a busy ED, it is important to understand not only the person's physical health needs but also the impact and stress an unplanned urgent admission can have on the individual and their family carers.

As highlighted in the case study by Melissa and Alexa, EDs are typically busy, at times chaotic, and are places that support people of all ages with various stages of distress and illness. Many EDs are not suitably designed for older adults in general but a person with dementia may find the environment particularly difficult. Events can happen fast in ED, which may make it more distressing for a person with a cognitive impairment, such as dementia. Constant stimulation from the noises of other patients in pain, machines beeping, and the movement and bustle of people in and out of rooms and cubicles can lead to an increase in distress behaviour exhibited by a person with dementia. In this environment a person with dementia may not be able to fully process what is happening around them. Many ED environments have been described as not being conducive to meeting older peoples' essential needs, particularly around providing continence care, identifying and managing pain, nutrition, and keeping the patient safe and comfortable (Dresden et al. 2022). Long waits on trollies can cause discomfort for people of any age, and in people with dementia this discomfort and the unfamiliar environment can lead to distress behaviours that staff may find difficult to manage.

ASSESSING THE PATIENT

Staff working in ED must remember that each person's experience of dementia will be different; what works for one person may not be useful for another. The impact of an admission to the ED can be overwhelming for the patient. During the health assessment the person with dementia may be unable to answer questions or have difficulty following even simple directions and requests.

The staff member carrying out the assessment needs to consider how the surroundings and assessment process may impact on the person with dementia, allow more time in asking their assessment questions and give the person more time to both process the information and then to reply. Melissa and Alexa identified that often ED staff are in the situation where they don't have access to a family member to give or corroborate information, and this can impede their assessment and care of the person with dementia. Attempts should be made to contact the family carer and, if possible, arrange for them to attend the ED to help with the assessment process should the patient have difficulty with communication.

Ideally, the assessment should be carried out in a quiet and calm area, with as few interruptions and distractions as possible to enable the person with dementia to achieve the best possible communication. Also check that the person has a hearing aid that is clean and working (if used) and clean glasses available (if worn) to enhance their ability to respond. Always ask what the patient needs, actively listen to those needs and clarify what has been said carefully and clearly; sometimes 'mirroring back' what they have said helps in clarifying what they say (Pepper and Harrison Dening, 2023). Always explain what is happening and is going to happen at each step of the process. You may need to repeat this, especially as short-term memory may be impaired.

Wherever possible, aim for consistency in having one member of staff completing the assessment and supporting the person during their time in the ED to aid continuity and for a rapport to be built. Be mindful of the possible negative impact of moving the person to different areas in the ED and try to limit this where possible. Ideally try and place the person with dementia in an area of the department that is closer to the nursing station so any distress can be quickly identified and managed. Also, they may find it comforting to have the nursing staff in their view.

When assessing a person with dementia, it is important to avoid interpreting any behaviours as being due to their dementia diagnosis. There is a risk that this 'diagnostic overshadowing' (Canevelli et al. 2016) can lead to the person not receiving the right care because the dementia diagnosis takes precedence above other conditions that they may present with or struggle to articulate. The assessor should be aware that distress can also be caused, or exacerbated, by physical issues such as pain, delirium, dehydration, infection and constipation. The person with dementia may not understand what is happening to them, or that the experience they are having is due to pain or an injury, and so respond with distressed behaviours. The root cause of their behaviours, such as pain, discomfort or ill health, should be investigated and then treated accordingly.

SUPPORTING FAMILY CARERS

The Dementia Friendly Hospital Charter (Dementia Action Alliance 2018) encourages partnership working with carers, supporting the person with dementia to enable choice and control over their care and appropriate support whilst attending hospital and on discharge. The charter recommends various interventions to do this in practice which includes organizational policies on carers, flexible visiting, assessment of patient and carer needs and use of initiatives which promote the rights of carers in hospital care such as John's Campaign (Gerrard and Jones 2017).

Melissa and Alexa recognized the importance of family carer involvement in their case study and indicated that they followed the principles of John's Campaign in their clinical practice. John's Campaign was founded by two carers following their personal experiences of the negative impact of hospital admissions and visiting restrictions on their loved ones. John's Campaign fights for the right of people living with dementia to be supported by their informal carers during hospital admission, to maintain wellbeing and prevent delirium, describing the role of carers as essential. The founders of John's Campaign highlight the impact of not involving informal carers and argue that not to do so means that an essential part of the support team is lost, making the delivery of care harder and more stressful for people with dementia and the care staff (Gerrard and Jones 2017). Further to this, they argue that the family carer also loses, as they will have to manage the decline and consequences of this distress and deconditioning following hospital attendance of the person with dementia.

To summarize, working in partnership with family carers, supporters and friends of a person with dementia in the ED supports improved experience and outcomes for all involved, including professionals.

PERSON-CENTRED APPROACH

Person-centred care is a term commonly used in nursing practice, policy and guidance and is considered a best practice approach to dementia care (Baillie and Thomas 2020). The value of adopting person-centred approaches in dementia care was pioneered by Kitwood in the 1990s who championed the importance of acknowledging the personhood of people with dementia, by seeing the person first (Kitwood and Brooker 2019). He defined personhood as one's status as a human being within society and relationships, which demands recognition, respect and trust.

Personal profiles, or personal information documents, support staff to deliver person-centred care through understanding individual needs and preferences when individuals with dementia are unable to communicate these themselves. They are often a short document, not an exhaustive or complex list of needs, and tend to focus on daily activities and preferences that a new staff member can quickly read to gain an understanding of some basic information. For example, preferred name with which to address the person, likes and dislikes, and useful approaches to reduce distress. Their purpose is having such preferences and needs briefly stated in a format that moves with the individual and is accessible to staff. A study by Clark et al. (2022) identified that having access to such a document to inform staff led to higher-quality care, reduced carer stress and improved communication, which they suggest all decrease avoidable morbidity and mortality. In a busy ED there often isn't time to start a detailed person-centred care plan, but some understanding of the person is essential to help prevent or manage distress whilst in the ED. Any information that is gathered in the ED could be recorded for the future care needs of the person with dementia, especially if they are admitted to a ward within the hospital.

CONSENT AND CAPACITY

Staff in busy EDs must always be aware of the principles of the Mental Capacity Act (MCA) when caring for people with dementia and remember that a diagnosis of dementia does not automatically mean the person lacks capacity for all decisions. The MCA aims to promote and safeguard decision making within a legal framework which ensures that vulnerable people are empowered to make decisions for themselves wherever possible and protects those who lack capacity. The MCA (2005) outlines five key principles:

- presumption of capacity
- the person being supported to make their own decisions
- a person has the right to make unwise decisions
- any decision made on a person's behalf should always be in the person's best interests
- least restrictive option for the person.

Therefore, when any decisions about care and treatment need to be made, staff should be mindful of these principles and document that they have assessed the patient's capacity for the specific decision.

CONCLUSION

EDs can be noisy, brightly lit and chaotic places and people who have dementia may be adversely affected by this and show signs of distress in addition to their presenting physical health problems. Resources in a busy ED are often stretched and this may lead to staff missing the early signs of distress in people with dementia when behaviours that ultimately challenge care can be prevented, reduced and effectively managed before they escalate. Prevention is better than cure, and in this chapter the Admiral Nurse details actions that can be taken to reduce the distress of people with dementia in the ED.

SOURCES OF SUPPORT

If you have any questions about helping a person with any aspect of dementia, call our free Helpline on 0800 888 6678 or email at helpline@dementiauk.org
If you would prefer a pre-booked appointment by phone or video, call via the Dementia UK website: www.dementiauk.org

RESOURCES

John's Campaign. https://johnscampaign.org.uk

REFERENCES

Baillie, L. & Thomas, N. (2020) Personal information documents for people with dementia: Healthcare staff's perceptions and experiences. *Dementia.* 19(3): 574–589.

Canevelli, M., Valletta, M., Trebbastoni, A. et al. (2016) Sundowning in dementia: Clinical relevance, pathophysiological determinants, and therapeutic approaches. *Frontiers of Medicine.* 3: 73. https://doi:10.3389/fmed.2016.00073

Clark, E., Wood, F. & Wood, S. (2022) Barriers and facilitators to the use of personal information documents in health and social care settings for people living with dementia: A thematic synthesis and mapping to the COM-B framework. *Health Expectations.* 25(4): 1215–1231.

Dementia Action Alliance (2018) *Dementia-friendly hospital charter.* www.dementiaaction.org.uk/assets/0003/9960/DEMENTIA-FRIENDLY_HOSPITAL_CHARTER_2018_FINAL.pdf

Dresden, S.M., Taylor, Z., Serina, P. et al. (2022) Optimal Emergency Department care practices for persons living with dementia: A scoping review. *Journal of the American Medical Directors Association.* 23(8): 1314.e1-1314.e29.

Gerrard, N. & Jones, J. (2017) The role and importance of carers in hospital. In: J. James, B. Cotton, J. Knight, R. Freyne, J. Petit & L. Gilby (Eds.), *Excellent dementia care in hospitals: A guide to supporting people with dementia and their carers.* London: Jessica Kingsley Publishers.

Kitwood, T. & Brooker, D. (2019) *Dementia reconsidered revisited: The person still comes first.* Open University Press: Berkshire, UK.

Manning, S.N. (2021) Managing behaviour that challenges in people with dementia in the Emergency Department. *Emergency Nurse.* 29(3): 34–40.

Mental Capacity Act (2005) www.legislation.gov.uk/ukpga/2005/9/introduction

Pepper, A. & Harrison Dening, K. (2023) Person-centred communication with people with dementia. *Nursing Older People*. https://doi.org/10.7748/nop. 2023. e1430

Poblador-Plou, B., Calderón-Larrañaga, A., Marta-Moreno, J. et al. (2014) Comorbidity of dementia: A cross-sectional study of primary care older patients. *BMC Psychiatry*. 14(1): 1–8.

CHAPTER 10

Nursing people with dementia in an acute ward

SOME OF THE DAY-TO-DAY CHALLENGES

INTRODUCTION

People with dementia are more likely to be admitted to an acute hospital ward for management of another co-morbid medical illness, rarely for diagnosis or management of dementia itself. An admission to an acute hospital, whether this be in the Emergency Department or to a hospital ward, can be unsettling for a person with dementia. As well as the fact the person is likely to be feeling unwell, it can also be disruptive to their usual routines, and this often results in distress (BGS 2022). Whilst every effort must be made to provide care that is person-centred and sensitive to the needs of people with dementia, there are many challenges to enabling this. The examples below provided by nurse Ella Balmer demonstrate some of the difficulties that can be experienced by nurses in caring for people with dementia on their wards. Following this a specialist dementia nurse (Admiral Nurse) explores how to provide care for people with dementia in an acute setting.

Ella Balmer, Enhanced Care and Support Nurse

There are many challenges for acute hospital nurses in providing care to their patients with dementia. One of the biggest challenges is in providing safe staffing levels when caring for patients living with dementia. At times it can feel like wards have an increasing number of patients who require one-to-one care than there are staff to deliver this intense level of support. Some acute hospitals have established teams of nurses who can advise ward staff how to work more effectively with patients with dementia and those with complex needs, for example supporting them in finding triggers for behaviours that challenge care delivery.

Encouraging patients with dementia to accept medications can also be a big challenge; as nurses we know how important mental health medications are to our patients. Finding alternative routes and returning multiple times to patients to assist them in taking medications can be very time consuming for nursing staff and distressing for our patients.

As a nurse I have noticed the inherently noisy hospital ward environment can be a trigger for some behaviours in our patients with dementia. Hospital wards are naturally busy places, and there are often around 26 patients on a ward all requiring their needs to be met. This often means that patients with dementia can become over-stimulated by the noise which can then lead to them presenting with agitation and becoming aggressive towards nursing staff.

Finally, a challenge we face relates to language barriers. We have had patients with dementia from black, minority and ethnic groups who have reverted to speaking in their native language, or patients who have never learnt to speak English. These issues on top of their dementia can cause distress for both patients and families. We try to accommodate this on the ward and allow relatives to translate for nursing staff. For some, the Enhanced Care nurses try to facilitate the use of picture cards where appropriate.

Kerry Lyons, Consultant Admiral Nurse
for Physical Health and Frailty

IMPROVING CARE FOR PEOPLE LIVING WITH DEMENTIA ON ACUTE WARDS

Ella refers to a range of challenges faced by acute nurses when caring for a person with dementia. Hospital admission for some people living with dementia can lead to increased confusion and escalated distress, which can have a negative impact on length of hospital stay, their usual ability and functional baseline, and their eventual care needs on discharge.

Ella referred to increasing numbers of patients with dementia within her hospital setting; currently one in four adult inpatient beds are occupied by a person with dementia, and these patients are six times more likely to experience an inpatient episode of delirium resulting in greater levels of confusion, distress and challenges to care delivery (NHS RightCare 2017).

It is important for hospitals to be able to reflect a commitment for continuous improvement of dementia care for patients and their families. This should include having resources and governance structures in place which support staff to deliver informed and high-quality dementia care (Dewing and Dijk 2016).

Many hospitals have introduced Enhanced Care and Support nurses such as Ella and her team to offer a specialist one-to-one resource and service to patients and their families, ensuring that ward staff have access to additional trained individuals who can use their specialist dementia knowledge to advise, undertake person-centred assessments, plan care and deliver focused interventions.

EDUCATION AND TRAINING

Dementia awareness education programmes should be embedded within all hospitals, to enable care staff to gain a greater understanding of the degenerative disease processes occurring within dementia, with an aim to promote a better understanding of individual need, and the importance of undertaking holistic assessments and person-centred care planning (Kitwood 1997). There is a wide range of dementia education packages currently available (Smith et al. 2019). Health Education England proposed a Three-Tiered Dementia Training Standards Framework, which articulates the knowledge and skills required for the health and social care workforce to deliver excellent quality dementia care. Many hospitals deliver Care Certificate training, incorporating dementia care as a core requirement for all healthcare support workers. In addition to this, most hospitals now offer basic dementia awareness e-learning education modules to all staff.

A core aspect of Ella's role is that of role modelling best practice – demonstrating to ward staff the importance of understanding a person's behaviour and possible reasons for this, alongside actively looking for ways in which to enhance and improve inpatient experience for both the patient and their carer. This form of education can have a positive effect on staff attitude, care culture, confidence in care delivery and knowledge of the disease process and symptom management; all of which can directly influence better care provision and outcomes. There are a number of hospitals which have appointed dementia-trained staff into the role of a dementia champion, which can be an enabler to share best practice within teams at all levels. In such cases, the dementia champions will have undertaken enhanced dementia training to improve their knowledge in delivering high-quality dementia care and support.

Training and education should also not 'just' cover dementia, but ideally also include prevention, identification and management of inpatient delirium, as dementia and delirium are often experienced together. All healthcare professionals should be familiar and competent with the use of validated standardized screening tools for the identification of both dementia and delirium. In addition to this, they should be aware of the potential underlying causes of delirium which are unmanaged pain, infection, disrupted sleep pattern, environmental factors, constipation, reduced nutrition and hydration, polypharmacy and harm (intentional; surgical or unintentional; inpatient fall or other harm) (Morandi et al. 2017).

UNDERSTANDING DELIRIUM

Understanding the symptoms of delirium can help to prevent, spot and stop further progression; being able to do this will certainly help to improve outcomes for patients with dementia. Understanding how to prevent future delirium can also be an important aspect in supporting a person and their family to live well with dementia. There is an increased risk of developing delirium in people with a history of dementia, depression, previous delirium, diseases causing cerebral irritation, abnormal metabolism and surgical interventions, as well as towards the end of life.

Delirium is sometimes difficult to recognize in patients with dementia because it has similar symptoms, for example memory impairment, disorganized thinking, misinterpretation, hallucinations (particularly visual) and personality changes. This can lead to a risk of mistaking delirium as advancing symptoms of dementia, and consequently delaying diagnosis and treatment of the condition. Recognizing early changes to a person's usual baseline can help to speed up the assessment and treatment process.

Indicators to look out for in a patient with delirium are:

- recent changes in cognitive function

- sudden increases in confusion

- visual or auditory hallucinations

- reduced movement

- restlessness and/or agitation

- social behaviour changes, such as a lack of cooperation or withdrawal.

When assessing changes to a patient's baseline, it is important to involve family carers, as they know the person living with dementia best of all and therefore are perfectly placed to see early changes in behaviour.

DISTRESSED BEHAVIOURS THAT CAN CHALLENGE CARE DELIVERY

Try to observe and understand changes in the person's behaviour, such as repetitive speech, repetitive actions, pacing, walking with purpose (often referred to as wandering), fidgeting and restlessness, agitation, sleep disturbance, apathy and disinterest; these are often ways a person with dementia is trying to express a need. These behaviours are often not a symptom of dementia, and represent distress due to frustration, unfamiliarity with a strange environment, increasing anxiety, unmanaged pain (physical or emotional) or fear.

Understanding a person's usual baseline, alongside their abilities, likes and dislikes can help to identify the underlying triggers which may be contributing to new and emerging behaviours. As professionals we need to be reframing these as 'distressed behaviours', rather than challenging behaviours.

Recording changes in behaviour on records such as ABC (Antecedents, Behaviour, Consequences) charts can help to identify circumstances around the person's behavioural change; noting factors prior to, during and after events. Reviewing behavioural records which clearly and chronologically describe a series of events in detail can offer vital clues and opportunities on how we can modify any triggers (both external and internal) that may be contributing to the person's distressed behaviours (NICE 2018).

Behaviour changes can result from a host of triggers:

- environment (unfamiliarity, increased noise, temperature, lighting)
- contact (interventions such as washing and dressing, continence support, dressing changes)
- time (early and/or end of the day episodes of confusion)
- underlying physical health issues (such as, delirium, pain or infection).

Actions to consider that may help:

- Offer reassurance.
- Create a quiet environment and/or quiet space – consider any risks if you choose a single room over a multiple bedded room.
- Consider using distraction techniques, meaningful engagement and activity.
- Personalize spaces wherever possible to encourage familiarity.

PRACTICAL GUIDANCE IN SUPPORTING A PATIENT EXPERIENCING INCREASED CONFUSION
Early identification
Seek early expert support to identify problem(s) and treat cause(s) of any increased confusion, ensuring early exclusion of delirium. It is important to involve carers at the earliest opportunity, as they will

often be key in identifying potential triggers and solutions (remember that they often know the person best of all).

Considerations for the patient's environment

Try to keep the environment familiar to the person to aid orientation; re-orientating with environmental cues can be helpful (notes, clocks, radio, verbal reassurance, etc.). Promote a good waking and sleep routine, consider the impact of lighting, noise and setting the scene for sleep at night-time.

Thinking about communication

Give time and space for communication. To aid communication, wherever possible minimize background noise. Think carefully about your positioning, so you are not sat too close, or standing over the person in an intimidating manner.

Address a person by their name, using a range of communication techniques: non-verbal (gestures, body language and, if appropriate, touch), talk clearly and calmly, breaking down simple tasks and offering ongoing reassurance. Use communication tools where appropriate such as a memo board, cue cards or picture/icon boards.

Consider potential language barriers, and the use of 'impartial' language interpretation (either a family member or hospital interpretation service or a combination of both depending on the purpose of the communication). It is important to note that a person's first language may not be English, and as dementia progresses, a person may revert partially or fully back to their mother tongue. Encourage the wearing of functioning hearing aids and clean spectacles to aid communication.

Routine and independence

Promote independence wherever possible (within their usual and current capabilities) to reduce deconditioning. Support the person to eat and drink at regular intervals (offering liked food and drink), and encourage good oral hygiene and the wearing of dentures (as appropriate to need).

MANAGING FALSE BELIEFS
(DELUSIONS AND ILLUSIONS)

It is important to be non-confrontational about false beliefs (delusions and illusions) (see Resources section), offering support and reassurance alongside acting to re-orientate the person. Acknowledge any distress by validating the person's feelings and give more time where there is increased confusion, which is associated with delirium. Reassure and involve carers and ensure clear lines of communication and regular updates on the care of the person with dementia.

BASELINES AND COLLATERAL HISTORY

Ensuring an accurate assessment of a patient's baseline and presenting need is critical to ensuring good-quality care delivery for patients and their families. It can offer an early opportunity to engage carers in care delivery by facilitating and understanding their needs also. As part of routine practice, the following key information about the person living with dementia should be recorded on admission:

- baselines – usual routines and abilities

- capacity

- delirium history

- Lasting Power of Attorney status

- frailty status

- cultural, religious and spiritual needs

- nutritional status

- communication ability

- history of current and previous needs

- personal history

- assessment of pain

- key people involved and contact details

- mobility assessment and falls risk

- medications.

The above items should be regularly reassessed during the patient's inpatient stay to identify any positive or negative shifts in the person's baseline.

There is a wide body of evidence to support the value of introducing support tools such as 'This Is Me' which can be used effectively to inform person-centred care delivery, enabling the most appropriate and least restrictive options to care delivery. It is important to remember that assessments undertaken should be reflective of the needs and wellbeing of both the patient and their carer (Biglieri 2018).

ENHANCING THE HEALING ENVIRONMENT

The environment in which we deliver care can make a significant impact to both the patient and their carer. There are a range of assessment tools and design principles that can be applied to a hospital setting (The King's Fund 2020). As Ella discussed, inpatient stays can be extremely challenging for patients with dementia, where the person may struggle to adapt to the busy, loud, unfamiliar and over-stimulating environment of an acute ward (Riquelme-Galindo and Lillo-Crespo 2021). The length of stay for a person with dementia is often almost double compared to older people without dementia, therefore getting the ward environment right can have a positive effect on their experience and clinical outcomes. Environmental considerations can also assist in reducing risks of harm, illness and deterioration leading to protracted lengths of hospital stay and associated care costs. Setting the ward scene for sleep promotion at night by encouraging usual sleep patterns, darkened bed spaces, changing into nightwear, low noise and limiting stimulation can help to promote wellness and healing.

There are a range of dementia-friendly hospital initiatives that are 'environmental specific', such as:

- introduction of communal spaces to encourage social interaction, stimulation and meaningful engagement (additionally these may be supported by the introduction of Enhanced Care teams and Care and Support nurses, like Ella's role, providing expert staffing resource to deliver meaningful engagement and activity programmes)

- reduction of moves and out-of-hours transfers for people with dementia

- dementia identification schemes that inform placement and observation of patients within ward settings

- enhanced signage and orientation cues around the ward and broader hospital site to improve wayfinding

- noise reduction schemes – introduction of quiet spaces.

SENSORY ABILITIES

As Ella stated, over-stimulating environments can pose a challenge to a person with dementia. An understanding of the effect of dementia on a person's sensory abilities, and how this may manifest in the patient struggling to differentiate between simultaneous sensory stimulations, can enable hospital staff to have a greater appreciation of the issues people with dementia face. Sensory overload contributes to increased confusion within inpatient settings. Impaired cognition can lead to heightened states of disorientation, poor time perception and related distressed behaviour. Enhancing the healing environment therefore is more than a consideration of 'just' the physical environment; it should always involve a holistic assessment, in terms of usual baselines, presenting and future care needs – all undertaken within a multi-disciplinary team approach (Hung et al. 2017).

LEAST RESTRICTIVE APPROACHES TO CARE

All hospitals should have a non-concordance policy in place, to guide actions if a person refuses care and treatment; the document will be underpinned by legal and ethical processes, i.e., the Mental Capacity Act for capacity assessment and best interest decisions and the Deprivation of Liberty Safeguards.

All interventions should:

- take a least restrictive approach (meaningful, non-custodial and person-centred)

- involve discussions with carers

- be clearly documented

- be regularly reviewed (involving multi-disciplinary team discussion where appropriate).

Involving family carers as early as possible can inform the team of important routines, triggers and interests, which can help to anchor a person with dementia to their unfamiliar environment, reducing any potential related distress (NHS RightCare 2017).

WORKING IN PARTNERSHIP WITH FAMILIES

When staff are overstretched, family carers can often experience poor and fragmented communication. Ensuring that family carers have access to specialist dementia support (such as an Admiral Nurse) can have a positive and significant impact (Aldridge 2019).

There are a range of ways in which hospitals can improve their carer support (NICE 2018):

- Introduce carer cards and carer passports.

- Introduce a hospital carer policy, demonstrating organizational strategic priorities around partnership in care with carers.

- Have processes in place to involve carers early, ensuring that care staff work triadically with carers as partners in care – this should include aspects of discharge care planning which starts at the earliest opportunity.

- Have processes in place to involve carers in the completion of baseline assessment and collateral history taking, ensuring the right information is recorded and understood.

- Support the principles of John's Campaign and be able to confidently advocate for the needs of families living with dementia (see Resources section). Ensure visiting practice reflects individual need, with reasonable adjustments made where possible.

- Introduce communication strategies for carers to help to keep them fully informed.

- Always include carers within the decision-making process, with acknowledgement that they are key stakeholders in care planning and delivery.

CONCLUSION

There are a wide range of actions that hospitals and the care team can undertake that will go some way to building an infrastructure to enable a better inpatient experience, care delivery and clinical outcomes for families affected by dementia.

SOURCES OF SUPPORT

If you have any questions about helping a person with any aspect of dementia, call our free Helpline on 0800 888 6678 or email at helpline@dementiauk.org
If you would prefer a pre-booked appointment by phone or video, call via the Dementia UK website: www.dementiauk.org

RESOURCES

John's Campaign. For the right to stay with people with dementia; for the right of people with dementia to be supported by their family carers. https://johnscampaign.org.uk
Dementia UK information leaflets. www.dementiauk.org/get-support/resources/our-leaflets/?gclid=CjwKCAjw-vmkBhBMEiwAlrMeFzoksoc86xLzzW_a-buq g88UzDiioRdetiDXnvb9YR1r6rWYkCoHCxoCoOkQAvD_BwE
Dementia UK. False beliefs and delusions in dementia. www.dementiauk.org/information-and-support/health-advice/false-beliefs-and-delusions-in-dementia

REFERENCES

Aldridge, Z. (2019) Supporting families and carers of people with dementia. In K. Harrison Dening (Ed.), *Evidence-based practice in dementia for nurses and nursing students.* London: Jessica Kingsley Publishers.
Biglieri, S. (2018) Implementing dementia-friendly land use planning: An evaluation of current literature and financial implications for greenfield development in suburban Canada. *Planning Practice & Research.* 33(3): 264–290.
British Geriatric Society (BGS) (2022) *BGS position statement: Person-centred acute hospital care for people with dementia.* www.bgs.org.uk/resources/bgs-position-statement-person-centred-acute-hospital-care-for-people-with-dementia
Dewing, J. & Dijk, S. (2016) What is the current state of care for older people with dementia in general hospitals? A literature review. *Dementia.* 15(1): 106–124.

Hung, L., Phinney, A., Chaudhury, H. et al. (2017) 'Little things matter!' Exploring the perspectives of patients with dementia about the hospital environment. *International Journal of Older People Nursing.* 12(3): e12153. https://doi:10.1111/opn.12153

The King's Fund (2020) *Environmental assessment tools.* https://www.worcester.ac.uk/about/academic-schools/school-of-allied-health-and-community/allied-health-research/association-for-dementia-studies/ads-consultancy/the-kings-fund-environmental-assessment-tools/home.aspx

Kitwood, T. (1997) *Dementia reconsidered: The person comes first.* London: Open University Press.

Morandi, A., Davis, D., Bellelli, G. et al. (2017). The diagnosis of delirium superimposed on dementia: An emerging challenge. *Journal of the American Medical Directors Association.* 18(1): 12–18.

National Institute for Health and Care Excellence (NICE) (2018) *Dementia: Assessment, management and support for people living with dementia and their carers (NG97).* www.nice.org.uk/guidance/ng97

NHS RightCare (2017) *NHS RightCare scenario: Getting the dementia pathway right.* www.england.nhs.uk/publication/gettingthe-dementia-pathway-right

Smith, S.J., Parveen, S., Sass, C. et al. (2019) An audit of dementia education and training in UK health and social care: A comparison with national benchmark standards. *BMC Health Service Research.* 19: 711. https://doi.org/10.1186/s12913-019-4510-6

Riquelme-Galindo, J. & Lillo-Crespo, M. (2021) Developing a dementia inclusive hospital environment using an Integrated Care Pathway design: Research protocol. *PeerJ.* 9:e11589. https://doi.org/10.7717/peerj.11589

Distress behaviours in 'live-in' domiciliary care

INTRODUCTION

People with dementia and their families often choose to have 24 hour care delivered in their own home rather than have an admission to a long-term care facility (Pollock et al. 2021). In these situations, live-in care is available through domiciliary care providers and is usually arranged privately. According to a study by Pollock et al. (2021) family carers most value the companionship, emotional and social support, and reliability from such domiciliary services. The advantages of 'live-in' care are that the person with dementia remains in their own familiar surroundings, there is dedicated one-to-one care, continuity of professional carers, the family carer is supported to continue providing home care, it can be cost effective, and the lifestyle of the person and pets can be accommodated. However, there are some disadvantages that need to be taken into consideration by families including the cost of any home modifications, space (a bedroom is required for the carer), reduced privacy for the person with dementia and any family members living with them, and lack of funding support (although Continuing Health Care funding can be obtained in some circumstances to help cover costs).

The two scenarios below provide an account of how Serenity, a professional 'live-in' carer, supported Andre, a person with dementia, with his personal hygiene and nutritional needs in his own home. Following this a specialist dementia nurse (Admiral Nurse) responds with advice on what to do when supporting a person with dementia, their spouse and the 'live-in' professional carer.

Serenity Underhill, Professional Carer, The Good Care Group

Andre has been living with Alzheimer's disease for a few years now. He is supported at home by his wife and a live-in carer. Andre is no longer able to walk and is looked after predominantly in bed, with some periods sitting out in his wheelchair and armchair each day. Andre relies on his carer to meet all his personal care needs; he is doubly incontinent and can no longer meet his own personal care needs. He also requires full support to eat and drink.

Scenario 1

When anyone approaches Andre to give him a wash or change his clothes or continence pad, he can often become very distressed. He frequently cries out 'ouch' at the gentlest of contact, or even when water touches him. He can present with behaviours that challenge a carer, such as lashing out or trying to grab them by the arm or hand and bend their fingers back. Andre is still quite strong so this can be very hard to manage. He will shout and swear at his wife and carers, calling us all sorts of names. All of these behaviours are ways of telling us that he is scared or confused by what is happening and does not understand what we are trying to do for him. Andre becomes more confused if there is more than one voice in the room; even that can become too much for him. He will frequently shout at us to 'Shut up! Too much talking!' This makes it difficult to explain to Andre what needs to happen and what we are about to do for him. Moving and handling with Andre can also be hard because he does not want to move or be moved. This is unavoidable when it comes to helping him to dress, undress, change his continence pad or when transferring him to his wheelchair or armchair. He becomes distressed and will frequently push backwards with his hips and upper body when rolled on his side. He will also try to grab and pinch anyone who tries to move him.

Where we can, we try to explain what is happening and give Andre time to take this in and calm down before re-approaching him. At times when this is unavoidable, such as halfway through a pad change, we use a very gentle tone and give him lots of reassurance that we aim to be as quick as we can. We try to help Andre to feel safe and secure and explain what we are doing at every stage.

Scenario 2

At mealtimes Andre needs full support. He swallows well and used to enjoy a wide variety of different foods. However, in the last six months Andre has begun to turn his head away, or clamp his lips tightly shut when prompted to eat or drink. This is often accompanied by shouting at his carer to hurry up and 'get on with it'. When offering Andre food, he will frequently say 'yes' then turn his head away and refuse to eat or drink what he had asked for. Conversely, Andre will say 'no!' then pop his mouth open ready to have a bite of toast or spoon of custard. When Andre eats, he has now started to 'pouch' each mouthful of food in his mouth. He will chew once or twice, then refuse to chew further and will simply shake his head when prompted to chew and swallow. This can be particularly worrying if Andre starts to fall asleep with food in his mouth in case he inhales this when more relaxed.

To overcome the challenges around refusing food and drink I mix up the textures, tastes and even temperatures of each bite so that Andre remains stimulated by what he is eating. This can seem strange but having something sweet and something savoury in alternating spoons works! Smaller meals and snacks, little and often also seem to help, as does giving Andre regular sips of water.

Dr Jane Pritchard, Consultant Admiral Nurse

Having a professional carer live in the house can be challenging for family members who may take some time to adjust to having another person, a stranger at first, living with them. The professional carer building a trusting, therapeutic relationship with family members is therefore of vital importance. Professional carers should take the time to get to know family members, to involve them in decision making, and to respect and value the contribution that they make towards the person with dementia's wellbeing, as experts about the person. Working as a team where family members are actively involved in the provision of care is important. Ryan et al. (2008) have argued that it is the relationships of the staff with not only the person with dementia but also the family carer that are central to their sense of purpose. Working as a professional carer can be extremely rewarding, and in

the 'Senses framework' Nolan et al. (2001) outlined how professionals can make a real difference to the lives of the family member and
the person with dementia through this partnership working. They
describe how relationships help to create a:

- sense of security – being confident in good care, support networks and timely help when needed, to be able to relinquish
  care when appropriate

- sense of continuity – to maintain shared pleasures/pursuits
  with the person with dementia, ensuring good standards of
  care maintained by others, to remain involved in care

- sense of belonging – maintaining valued relationships, confid-
  ing in others and feeling like they are not in this alone

- sense of purpose – maintaining wellbeing and personhood of
  family carers

- sense of achievement – developing new skills and abilities, to
  know that you have provided the best possible care and done
  your best

- sense of significance – to feel caring efforts are valued and
  appreciated; enhanced sense of self.

To overcome reduced privacy and feelings of intrusion it is always
important that professional carers respect that they are working in the
person's own home, and that they are a guest there. This is particularly
important for family members who will likely want time alone with
the person with dementia from time to time, maintaining a sense
of intimacy and meeting emotional needs relating to their relationship. This need should be anticipated, and sensitively managed by
the professional carer who should ensure that family members are
offered and even encouraged to take this time together, meaning that
the professional carer will need to withdraw, but still be available
if assistance is required. For professional carers, developing a close
relationship with the family may take time, and the most important
aspect of the relationship is building trust that the carer can be relied
upon to provide high-quality care, especially when the family member
leaves the house and they are alone with the person. This feeling

of being able to take time for themselves is especially important to family members, who value this time and need it to meet their own emotional, psychological and physical needs.

The relationship may be tested from time to time when there are differing opinions between professional carers and family members about what is in the person's best interests, and about exactly how care should be delivered. Clarifying roles and responsibilities at an early stage can help to avoid misunderstandings and potential conflict. Open dialogue, sharing of knowledge from both sides, and an appreciation of differing points of view is also important with live-in care to maintain good working relationships. Professional carers must always be aware however of professional boundaries, and the need to follow their training (moving and handling training for example) and local policies, seeking advice from their employer where conflicting opinions cannot be resolved.

The scenarios illustrate some of the complexities when providing care in a person's own home where carers may find themselves working alone, with other care agencies or alongside family caregivers. The home environment has advantages for the person with dementia in that it is more familiar and homely, but carers may also find themselves with space restrictions. When a person with dementia gets distressed, for example when receiving personal care, swapping to a different carer to complete the intervention can help to defuse the situation, but this is not possible when there is a sole live-in carer. In this situation rather than swapping staff for the intervention, the live-in carer could make sure the person with dementia is safe, then leave the room and return a short time afterwards to resume the intervention, providing time for the person to calm down.

In the study by Dalgarno and colleagues (2021), family carers were asked what they needed from professional carers, and they indicated that consistency of worker was important. The family carers who took part in the study also stated that it was important that the professional carer be able to adapt to the changing needs of the person with dementia and the family. With 'live-in' care there is the opportunity to really get to know the person with dementia and their family which provides the opportunity for personalized care and ongoing collaboration between all parties, as evidenced in the scenarios written by Serenity.

DISTRESS

Behavioural challenges can be particularly hard for a spouse or partner who lives with the person with dementia, who may feel that they have no respite from the behaviours, who may feel guilt when witnessing aggression towards professional carers and who may even be injured themselves. The role of the Admiral Nurse therefore often embraces supporting the professional carer(s) with the practical challenges they face, supporting the family member needing emotional support, and also supporting the person with dementia in trying to reduce the distress they experience.

PERSONAL CARE

An approach that can be tried during personal care involves identifying any areas of underlying unmet need. As personal care is often perceived as an invasive procedure it can invoke a fear response in the person with dementia, and thus a need for comfort and security, as well as a need for control over their own body. Giving the person as much control over the process as possible may be helpful, such as gently enabling and encouraging them to do as much as they can for themselves, even if this is simply washing a small part of their own body such as their face with prompting. The 'hand under hand' technique developed by Snow (2021) can be beneficial for this, where the professional carer places their own hand underneath that of the person with dementia, guiding the person's hand, and allowing the person to feel as if they are carrying out the task themselves, retaining a feeling of being in control. Providing the person with something to hold onto such as a dry flannel may also give them a feeling of control and something else to focus on. Care should be taken to keep the person warm to prevent discomfort, and reduce reluctance to engage in the task, with their modesty and dignity always preserved with warm towels. Some people with dementia dislike the feeling of water on their skin and head so this should be taken into consideration when thinking about personal hygiene products, such as foams which some people prefer. Some people prefer their hair to be washed with a jug whilst in the bath rather than during a shower or using a shower head attachment. Leave-in conditioners and shampoos and dry shampoos are also available to reduce the amount of water that is required. Comforting, familiar music could be played to see whether this helps to reduce distress at this time; some professional carers even find that singing along together helps to lighten the mood and build a trusting relationship.

PAIN AND DISCOMFORT

Pain is commonly a cause of reluctance to engage in personal care, and for distress and aggression towards professional carers, as the person can believe that the professional carer is causing the pain and deliberately trying to hurt them. Aggression towards others in these circumstances can be seen therefore as a form of self-defence, and a way of stopping the pain. People with dementia who are experiencing pain are less likely to be able to express this verbally which leads to pain often not being identified and treated (Jonsdottir and Gunnarsson 2021). If someone grimaces, holds part of their body, or makes vocalizations such as 'ouch', as in Andre's case, then pain is something that should be investigated and treated. Pain may be experienced only on moving, which needs to be taken into consideration and pre-empted with analgesia before personal care takes place. Non-verbal pain scales such as the Abbey Pain Scale (Abbey et al. 2004) and Pain Assessment in Advanced Dementia (PAINAD; Warden et al. 2003) can be used to identify pain in people with dementia who are unable to vocalize this for themselves. These are short and easy to complete, meaning that professional carers can carry this out themselves before and during episodes of personal care. A change between the scores is suggestive of pain on being moved. Monitoring of pain is needed in people with dementia who have conditions likely to cause pain and discomfort such as chronic wear on the spine (spondylosis), arthritis and shortening and tightening of muscles, tendons and joints causing contractures. These conditions are likely to worsen over time, so even when a person was not taking pain relief prior to their dementia diagnosis, the need for analgesia is likely to change along with their condition. Where a person is thought to be in pain during personal care, regular rather than 'as required' medications should be sought from their GP to ensure their comfort. Where people with dementia do not tolerate or cannot take oral medications, alternatives such as a pain patch can be explored with their prescriber. In some circumstances, where the person does not wish to take oral medications and they lack the mental capacity to make this decision for themselves, a best interest decision under the Mental Capacity Act (2005) may be taken that the medication is given covertly, with the agreement of all those involved in their care, in the person's best interests.

COMMUNICATION

When communicating with people with dementia, ensure that shorter sentences than normal are used, which are easier for the person to process and understand. Use a low, clear, calm tone of voice so that you do not sound anxious or stressed, emotions that could be noticed and mirrored by the person with dementia. If the person wears hearing aids or glasses make sure that they are clean and working (replace batteries on hearing aids regularly), as wearing these will ensure communication is as easy as possible, avoiding any misunderstandings, and so that the person can hear the reassurances that are given, and see the care staff more clearly, reducing feelings of fear. Calm, open and positive non-verbal body language is important to reassure the person that they are safe (see 'Tips for communication' in Resources, and Chapter 5 for more on communication).

EATING AND DRINKING

It is important to assess the eating patterns and nutritional intake of people with dementia as dementia can lead to difficulties with eating and drinking, including appetite changes, forgetting to eat or drink, weight loss and swallowing problems (Fostinelli et al. 2020). Where the person is reluctant to eat always investigate whether there are any tooth or gum issues that may be making eating difficult, checking the inside of the mouth regularly when brushing to help to rule this out as a cause. Offering favourite foods may persuade the person to eat, and consider whether the person has developed a 'sweet tooth' and would prefer fruit or sugar in cereal or porridge, for example. Sometimes people with dementia may find it easier to eat with their fingers rather than using cutlery, and so foods that the person can eat independently like toast or small sandwiches may be preferred to being fully assisted with eating by another person, which may be perceived as invasive and unwelcome.

CONCLUSION

People with dementia and their families want to remain at home in an environment where they feel safe and secure for as long as is possible. Live-in care in their own home is a solution for many families who have the resources and room in their house to accommodate this. The continuity of service and the relationship is often highly valued by families and the live-in carer enables the development of personalized care focused on the needs of the whole family.

SOURCES OF SUPPORT

If you have any questions about helping a person with any aspect of dementia, call our free Helpline on 0800 888 6678 or email at helpline@dementiauk.org
If you would prefer a pre-booked appointment by phone or video, call via the Dementia UK website: www.dementiauk.org

RESOURCES

Dementia UK. Tips for communication. www.dementiauk.org/get-support/ understanding-changes-in-dementia/tips-for-better-communication

REFERENCES

Abbey, J., Piller, N., Bellis, A.D. et al. (2004) The Abbey pain scale: A 1-minute numerical indicator for people with end-stage dementia. *International Journal of Palliative Nursing*. 10(1): 6–13.
Dalgarno, E.L., Gillan, V., Roberts, A. et al. (2021) Home care in dementia: The views of informal carers from a co-designed consultation. *Dementia*. 20(7): 2261–2277.
Fostinelli, S., De Amicis, R., Leone, A. et al. (2020) Eating behavior in aging and dementia: The need for a comprehensive assessment. *Frontiers in Nutrition*. 7: 604488.
Jonsdottir, T. & Gunnarsson, E.C. (2021) Understanding nurses' knowledge and attitudes toward pain assessment in dementia: A literature review. *Pain Management Nursing*. 22(3): 281–292.
Mental Capacity Act (2005) www.legislation.gov.uk/ukpga/2005/9/introduction
Nolan, M., Davies, S. & Grant, G. (Eds.) (2001) *Working with older people and their families: Key issues in policy and practice*. Buckingham: Open University Press.
Pollock, K., Wilkinson, S., Perry-Young, L. et al. (2021) What do family caregivers

want from domiciliary care for relatives living with dementia? A qualitative study. *Ageing & Society.* 41(9): 2060–2073.

Ryan, T., Nolan, M., Reid, D. et al. (2008) Using the senses framework to achieve relationship-centred dementia care services: A case example. *Dementia.* 7(1): 71–93.

Snow, T. (2021). *Bathing and dementia – with Teepa Snow of Positive Approach to Care (PAC).* www.youtube.com/watch?v=iKT9YIVPREE

Warden, V., Hurley, A.C. & Volicer, L. (2003). Development and psychometric evaluation of the Pain Assessment in Advanced Dementia (PAINAD) scale. *Journal of the American Medical Directors Association.* 4(1): 9–15.

CHAPTER 12

Community nursing

RESPONDING TO DISTRESS

INTRODUCTION

People with dementia often have other multiple long-term conditions in addition to their dementia that may require support from a community or district nursing team. Community nurses are often well placed to deliver person- and relationship-centred care to families affected by dementia (Harrison Dening and Hibberd 2016). Often for these families the community nurse may be the only professional with whom they have regular contact. The nurse has an important role in assessing changes to a person's condition over time, identifying difficulties and risks, and providing emotional support to both the person with dementia and their family carers. However, delivery of care to families affected by dementia can be challenging, particularly where the person with dementia has difficulty understanding the reasons for the community nursing input and treatment plan, or where there are distress behaviours during a visit. Some of these challenges are illustrated in the case study in this chapter, following which a specialist dementia nurse (Admiral Nurse) suggests ways that distress and communication difficulties can be overcome in the community setting.

Julie Bentham, District Nurse

As a nurse working in the community there are a number of challenges we experience when caring for a person with dementia. The challenges often start from the point of referral, when we receive only basic information about the person; for example, that the person needs their wound dressing and that they have a diagnosis of dementia. Only on entering the person's home can the extent of their confusion become apparent.

When the person is very confused the task of dressing the wound can often take longer than anticipated, as extra time may be required to explain to the person who we are and what we need to do before the treatment can commence. Sometimes, we even have to repeat this several times during the procedure.

Where dressing of a wound is required, we need to give careful consideration to the type of dressing we use and think about what the least restrictive option might be. For example, avoiding big and bulky dressings which are more likely to be removed if the person with dementia finds them uncomfortable.

Providing treatment involving dressings (or any treatments involving close physical contact) can be challenging if the person becomes distressed. Often this distress can come from the person forgetting what we are there for, or what we are doing, and this can result in the person with dementia grabbing, scratching or shouting at the nurse. To manage this, we need to have a calm approach, using continuous explanation to make sure the person understands what we are doing and why. This is made much easier when we are able to see the person daily, allowing a therapeutic relationship and trust to be built, both with the person with dementia and their family carers. It is also important that we follow the principles of person-centred care, tailoring care plans to each individual and building in extra time for communication.

Often as community nurses we are the first professionals to recognize when there is a risk present (for example safeguarding concerns, environmental, physical and mental health risks) for the person with dementia. Where risks are identified we will refer on to other agencies, for example mental health services, GP, safeguarding or social care.

Victoria Davies, Admiral Nurse

Julie's case study highlights some important issues faced by district nurses, many of which we recognize and are familiar with as Admiral

Nurses. This section will draw on Julie's case study to offer advice on supporting people with dementia and their families living in a community setting.

REFERRAL – GATHERING INFORMATION TO INFORM MANAGEMENT OF THE VISIT

As Julie highlights in her case study, challenges in the community nurse role can start from the point of referral, when only basic information about the person is given. Such a referral can be indicative of 'diagnostic overshadowing', where the emphasis is on the dementia and not the person. Every person with dementia will experience and manage their condition differently, and will have their own unique set of circumstances, including other health conditions, age, life history and current living situation, all of which are important to be aware of when planning their treatment at home, and in deciding what resources might be needed (for example how long is needed for the visit, and any equipment needed).

Person-centred care is about understanding the strengths, abilities and needs of the person (and their family carer) and being able to meet those identified needs with an individualized plan of care. When a referral lacks the necessary background detail to be able to understand a person's strengths and challenges, it makes it harder to practice in a person-centred way. It is therefore important to consider if more information is needed, either from the referrer, from other professionals involved in the person's care, from family carers or from the person themselves, prior to carrying out the visit.

RISK ASSESSMENT BEFORE VISITING

If there is concern about the person with dementia having a history of distress behaviours, either suggest a joint visit with the referrer or a member of a team who has been involved with the person. When you review a person's history there may be patterns that indicate known triggers of distress for them. For example, someone may be known to become distressed when a male nurse visits them. There may be religious or educational issues that impact on how you deliver care to the person with dementia. Review previous contact notes to see if there is any time of the day where visits have been more successful. This could enable the district nurse to plan in extra time for the visit and visit at a time of day when the person is likely to be more receptive to an intervention (Hoe et al. 2023).

It may also be helpful to find out if the person has had the same treatment or procedure in the past, how well they tolerated it and anything that helped them cope with it better. Armed with this information, you can acknowledge to the person that they have been through a similar procedure before and that it was managed with a good outcome. Demonstrating this level of knowledge of the person and their past treatments may be reassuring for them.

If deemed urgent and there is no background information provided in the referral, speak with the referrer to gain further understanding of the circumstances. In line with local policies, a risk assessment may need to be completed, and a decision made about whether the visit will require two people in attendance. In addition, it is advisable that work colleagues know where you are, with timings, when working in the community and to always consider exit routes in case of emergency.

MANAGING A VISIT WHEN THE PERSON WITH DEMENTIA LIVES ALONE

Many GP practices now use SMS texts to provide patients with information or appointment reminders (Sallis et al. 2019). Before visiting the person with dementia, text them with a reminder of your visit or call them directly, remembering to give your name and explaining your role. This will help to remind them of your impending visit. If the person is unable to use a phone, then find out if there is an identified family member or professional carer who the reminder can be sent to.

Be prepared to consider how you can effectively communicate and convey your messages at the door (see Table 12.1). People with dementia can experience visual distortions due to reflections, poor lighting and changes to their visual field. Ensure your professional identity card is easy to read – consider if you need a bigger print or a distinct contrasting background to make it easier for someone with dementia to read and understand.

Table 12.1: Preventing and managing potential risks in the community

Advice	Rationale
Have an open and friendly approach and be aware of maintaining personal space.	A person with dementia may feel distressed if they perceive that their personal space is invaded or that the body language of the person coming to their house is threatening.
Introduce yourself clearly and show means of identification and state the intention of the visit.	If the person with dementia doesn't know who is visiting and why, they will be more reluctant to let the person in.
If the person visited has a pet, consider whether to have them in the room whilst the intervention takes place.	For some people having their pets in the room can help them to feel more relaxed and less distressed when an intervention takes place. If the pet is likely to become distressed or interferes with the intervention this could be explained to the person and a request made to put it into another room or outside.
Pay attention to the person who is receiving an intervention and explain what is happening and why.	If the reason for the visit and intervention is not explained the person is more likely to become distressed and less likely to agree to take part in the intervention.
Reduce the number of distractions during the visit.	If the person with dementia thinks that the nurse visiting is ignoring them or takes calls during the visit, they are more likely to become distressed.
If the person visited has communication difficulties, find out what works for them, e.g., written instructions, cards with key words or pictures.	If the person with dementia has communication difficulties this can lead to a misunderstanding, frustration and distress, especially if the person visiting them does not acknowledge this or make suitable adaptations for their communication (see Chapter 5 for more on communication and dementia).

A person with dementia may not be able to give you verbal consent but may indicate their response via gestures. It is for this reason that plenty of time must be allowed for a person with dementia to demonstrate their consent or lack thereof to treatment. Another strategy could be to have a green (okay) card and red (stop) card which the person with a dementia can point to or hold up as you carry out the procedure. Using this approach, you can also ask the person a question and point to cards; this will help with clarity and provides assurances for them that you are listening. A similar approach can also be used if you are assessing for the presence of pain, for example by using a Visual Analogue Scale, which could be laminated and used to help rate pain.

Some common problems you may encounter at this point are discussed below.

The person has no recollection of your planned visit

This can happen even after you have sent an SMS text message or made a telephone call. Keep calm and maintain a relaxed posture. Explain the reason for your visit, ensuring you use language that is easy to understand, avoiding the use of clinical jargon. If you are attending to dress a wound, as in Julie's case study, you could try pointing out the position of the wound on your own body and verbally repeating the reason, or if you observe the area of the problem, you can point and remark, 'That's what I have come to help you with.'

Should the person with dementia continue to decline the visit, respect that decision. Advise that you will try again later and ask if there is a preferred time to call back. You could leave your written contact details with the date and time you called as a further prompt. By doing this, someone else such as a family member who visits the person may pick up the details and contact you. If you cannot follow through with the visit if the person with dementia continues to decline, advise the referrer. A solution could be a joint visit with you and the professional making the referral.

As Julie states, some people with dementia can find home visits, for things like wound dressings, difficult to cope with and may show signs of distress, such as shouting or pushing you away. The tips in Box 12.1 can help to prevent and manage distress.

Box 12.1: Preventing and managing distress as a community nurse performing a procedure

→ Advise the person with dementia that they can stop the procedure until they are happy to proceed again.

→ Take your time with the procedure and ideally break it

down into smaller tasks, asking at each stage if it is okay to continue.

→ Ask the person with dementia (and their carer if relevant) if they have had the procedure before, and if so, how did they cope with this?

→ Maintain a calm environment and keep distractions to a minimum.

→ Speak and behave in a calm and friendly manner and reassure the person with dementia if they are starting to get distressed, and pause the procedure until they feel able to continue again.

→ Observe for any non-verbal signs of discomfort and distress and pause the procedure until the person feels better able to cope.

→ If the person with dementia becomes distressed and the procedure needs to be stopped completely make sure they are comfortable before leaving them.

→ Make contact with the family carer and explain what happened and what the plans are to continue the procedure at a later date, and indicate whether or not their assistance may be required.

→ Report and record the lack of progress with the procedure and the associated distress displayed by the person with dementia, including, if possible, what caused the distress, what happened and how this was managed.

Person with dementia declines treatment

People with dementia may retain capacity to make treatment decisions. However, as the effects of their dementia increase their capacity can fluctuate and change. If you can understand the person and how they prefer to communicate and understand their specific circumstance, their ability to have agency over their decisions can be supported. If this is the case, then the person's decision should be clearly recorded in their notes and reported back to the referrer and any other relevant professionals.

Living with advanced dementia may result in the person lacking capacity to consent to treatment; in these cases a mental capacity assessment (MCA 2005) can be undertaken, specific to the decision to be made, and consideration given to how the procedure can be carried out in their best interests.

MANAGING A VISIT WHEN THE PERSON WITH A DEMENTIA HAS IDENTIFIED SUPPORT NEEDS

The person may have regular support of a family member or profes-sional carer. If you have arranged an appointment through a family member, they may answer the door which may give you a chance to talk to them alone. There may be things they want to tell you that they can't easily say in front of the person with dementia. When greeting, check in with them to see how things are and if there is anything you need to be aware of. Find out if there are any communication difficulties, such as hearing loss, visual problems or dysphasia that will influence your initial approach.

A complicated procedure or dressing might require the collabo-ration of the family carer to soothe and respond to the person with dementia. Discuss with the family member or carer what they need to do and check that they are comfortable with assisting you. Box 12.1 provides tips on preventing and managing distress when working with a person with dementia who needs an intervention.

OTHER CHALLENGES
Management of posture

People with dementia often experience changes to their proprio-ception (the body's ability to sense movement, action and location in the environment) which can affect how they understand their body's position. They may therefore have difficulty in maintaining the position of a limb, be prone to leaning, or may not be able to move a limb with ease. All these presentations may be perceived as distress behaviours when in fact they are due to the symptoms of dementia (Harrison Dening and Aldridge, 2021). Before carrying out a dressing procedure make sure that the person is sitting comfortably and that their posture is well supported. Feet should be firm on the floor and affected limbs supported by pillows or cushions. This helps the person with dementia to be comfortable whilst the procedure is taking place.

Management of dressings

Where you have applied a dressing to a person with dementia there are a few strategies to prevent them removing it when you have gone. This could include use of long sleeves or trousers to cover the dressed area. Depending on the type of wound dressing and its properties, either cover with a bandage or a sleeve of another elastic net dressing or elasticated tubular bandage. On some dressings you may be able to write a reminder on it advising the person not to remove, or even placing a small red cross on the dressing may prevent removal. Unfortunately, unless there is someone reminding them of the reason for the dressing, even if the above strategies are used, there may be occasions when the dressing is removed.

Risks identified at time of visit

If during the visit you have any concerns or risks become evident, such as being unable to carry out the treatment or observable self-neglect, these will need to be reported through safeguarding processes. Every locality has safeguarding teams and procedures to follow. At times this might make you feel conflicted as a nurse, however safeguarding is an important part of a nurse's role. Having identified a risk does not make you solely responsible for it – what is important is that all risks are reported via the proper local processes to make sure that the person is kept safe, and their wellbeing is maintained.

CONCLUSION

Reviewing and analysing the referral information you have access to and identifying any that is missing which would support the completion of your visit is important. To gain as much information as possible may also mean speaking directly with the person with dementia and their family members and carers beforehand to ensure

WHAT YOU *REALLY* WANT TO KNOW ABOUT WORKING WITH DEMENTIA

your approach is person-centred. The time spent on gaining the person's health history and how they have responded to treatments in the past will provide a good understanding of how to engage with them now. This will also give a much better understanding of any known risks and help in judging how much time is needed for the appointment and any specific communication strategies that might be needed (e.g., written notes, language, pictures).

Using professional curiosity to establish a better understanding of the home situation and strengths of the person with dementia may sound time consuming and might be viewed as unwieldy for a team that is likely to be under pressure. However, in the long term that effort is most likely to pay off with a positive outcome of a successful visit.

SOURCES OF SUPPORT

If you have any questions about helping a person with any aspect of dementia, call our free Helpline on 0800 888 6678 or email at helpline@dementiauk.org
If you would prefer a pre-booked appointment by phone or video, call via the Dementia UK website: www.dementiauk.org

RESOURCES

Dementia UK. **Pain and dementia.** www.dementiauk.org/wp-content/uploads/dementiauk-pain-and-dementia-leaflet-DUK27-2023.pdf
Dementia UK. **Frailty and dementia.** www.dementiauk.org/wp-content/uploads/dementia-uk-frailty.pdf
Dementia UK. **Keeping safe when you care for someone with dementia.** www.dementiauk.org/wp-content/uploads/dementia-uk-keeping-safe.pdf

REFERENCES

Harrison Dening, K. & Aldridge, Z. (2021) Understanding behaviours in dementia. *Journal of Community Nursing.* 35(3): 50–55.
Harrison Dening, K. & Hibberd, P. (2016) Exploring the community nurse role in family-centred care for patients with dementia. *British Journal of Community Nursing.* 21(4): 198–202.
Hoe, J., Trickey, A. and McGraw, C. (2023) Caring for people living with dementia in their own homes: A qualitative study exploring the role and experiences of registered nurses within a district nursing service in the UK. *International Journal of Older People Nursing.* 18(1): e12491.
Mental Capacity Act (2005) www.legislation.gov.uk/ukpga/2005/9/introduction

Sallis, A., Sherlock, J., Bonus, A. et al. (2019) Pre-notification and reminder SMS text messages with behaviourally informed invitation letters to improve uptake of NHS Health Checks: A factorial randomised controlled trial. *BMC Public Health*. 19: 1162. https://doi.org/10.1186/s12889-019-7476-8

CHAPTER 13

Driving and dementia

'LIFE WITHOUT A CAR...'

INTRODUCTION

Driving safely requires us to use a number of skills, including decision making, reacting quickly and our visuo-spatial skills. All of these are things that may be affected by dementia, and it is not uncommon for health and social care practitioners to become concerned that driving may present a risk to a person living with dementia (Wilson and Pinner 2013). Balancing risks was one of the key themes from our survey, and we know that giving up driving can have a huge impact on quality of life, presenting a dilemma for professionals as they seek to balance the risks to safety with the risks to a person's quality of life.

The case study below provides an account of how Alison, an occupational therapist, supported a family through the process of a memory assessment where there were also concerns about driving, and ultimately to thinking about 'life without a car'. Following this a specialist dementia nurse (Admiral Nurse) will respond with advice on what to do if you are concerned about someone's driving safety, how best to support families with these difficult conversations, the legal aspects of continuing to drive after a diagnosis and how to support families in adjusting to no longer being able to drive.

Alison Holden, Occupational Therapist,
Memory Assessment Service

Albert was a 77-year-old gentleman referred to the memory assessment service (MAS) by his GP with a 12-month history of memory difficulties which were starting to impact upon his day-to-day life. Aside from these memory difficulties, he was otherwise fit and healthy, with some mild arthritis and history of high blood pressure which was managed with medication. Albert was a retired postman and enjoyed various hobbies including going out to play bowls and attending local church activities with his wife. Albert still drove, and driving, to him, was more than just a means of transport; it was something he had always loved to do and enjoyed. His wife Kath did not drive, and mobility problems meant she could not walk very far outdoors. Their children lived locally, and they also had good support from neighbours.

Albert was visited at home for his initial MAS assessment and there was evidence of both cognitive and functional decline. Albert had difficulties across all domains including visuo-spatial problems. Albert did accept he had some difficulties with his memory but was not too concerned ('…it's just old age') and he felt this was not impacting on his function at all and certainly not his ability to drive. Kath was concerned both about his memory and his driving, stating that he had on occasion got lost when driving familiar routes and that there had been a couple of 'near misses' with other cars. The assessing clinician advised Albert to refrain from driving until his full assessment was completed, including a CT brain scan and seeing the MAS doctor.

Discussing Albert's driving clearly created conflict and tension in the couple. Albert was angry that this assessment could potentially lead to him losing his driving licence and was concerned about the impact this would have upon their freedom, independence and access to the activities they both enjoyed. 'How will we manage…?' 'How will we get to the supermarket, the church or visit our family…?'

Kath however expressed her relief that this issue was now being addressed by someone other than herself, although she was equally as worried about what this would mean for them, given she could not walk very far or drive herself. She was also worried about managing Albert's reaction to being advised to stop driving. The difficult feelings unearthed by the conversation on driving, as well as the differing views of Albert and Kath, felt difficult for the clinician involved to manage. They were concerned that despite providing all

DRIVING AND DEMENTIA: 'LIFE WITHOUT A CAR...'

the necessary clinical advice these discussions would impact upon the patient/clinician relationship, and that Albert would not continue with the full MAS assessment if it meant he may be advised to stop driving.

Nevertheless, six weeks later and following his CT brain scan Albert did come to clinic to see the MAS doctor. Albert was given a diagnosis of Alzheimer's dementia and advised by the doctor that he would need to inform the DVLA about his diagnosis and, as previously advised, to refrain from driving until the DVLA had made their decision on whether they would be revoking his licence. Albert was again quite angry as well as shocked with this outcome, an understandable reaction one could say, given he had received the diagnosis of dementia and the advice about driving cessation within the same appointment – a significant life transition for both Albert and his family. Kath was also upset but understood the reasons for these decisions and thanked the team for their support and guidance with regard to this issue so far. She reported that Albert never really thought this would happen but now they, as a family, would start to plan for the future and potentially 'life without a car'.

Joanne Freeman, Admiral Nurse, Admiral Nurse Dementia Helpline

DRIVING AND DEMENTIA

Driving is a complex task, requiring us to use a number of different skills and abilities, including memory, visuo-spatial skills, attention, concentration and our executive functions, all of which can be affected by dementia (Bennett 2022). This case study reflects a concern that is frequently voiced to Admiral Nurses by families undergoing assessment for dementia and following the diagnosis. As the case study highlights, often driving is more than just a mode of transport, it also has an emotional resonance that can represent independence, freedom and normality. Therefore, the thought of not being able to drive whilst in the process of getting a diagnosis can feel overwhelming and possibly lead to the person expressing anger, becoming distressed or even depressed (Holden and Pusey 2021). As clinicians this can be challenging, as we need to navigate the legal aspects of driving and dementia, initiate conversations about a person's own accountability to remain within the law and safe on the roads, and in many cases have difficult discussions about the cessation of driving (Holden and Pusey 2021).

HOW DEMENTIA IMPACTS ON DRIVING ABILITY

The damage caused to the brain by dementia can affect a person's ability to drive safely in a number of ways (see Box 13.1).

Box 13.1: How dementia affects driving ability

→ As memory becomes affected the person may become lost and struggle to recognize where they are; sometimes things that are familiar can become unrecognizable or unfamiliar which can be upsetting and disorientating. This can cause problems with remembering routes whilst driving.

→ Dementia can cause problems with spatial awareness such as the ability to judge distances which could make it difficult to park a car, and judge breaking distances and road positioning.

→ Decision making can also be affected which could result in people making poor or rash decisions when driving, and having difficulty understanding and reacting to the actions of other drivers.

→ Dementia can cause problems with focus and attention, which can make it more difficult to maintain focus on the different aspects of driving simultaneously.

→ When problem-solving skills are affected it can become more difficult for a person with dementia to cope with unexpected events whilst driving, for example another road user driving erratically, diversions or other obstacles such as pedestrians, cyclists or parked cars.

> → Reaction times can be impacted by dementia, and this
> poses an obvious risk in terms of being able to act quickly
> to avoid an accident.

Whilst all the above problems can be associated with a diagnosis of dementia, a person's functional ability in relation to driving will also be associated with the stage of their dementia. With a move towards earlier detection and diagnosis of dementia, it may be that a person who is recently diagnosed is able to continue driving for a period of time. Others who may be diagnosed in the later stages of dementia may have to stop driving straight away, as their functional impairment may indicate this as the best course of action.

THE LEGAL ASPECTS OF DRIVING AND DEMENTIA

Driving and dementia slightly differs to most of the advice we give; Admiral Nurses aim to problem solve and encourage people to live as independently as possible for as long as possible, encouraging both the person with dementia and their families to concentrate on what *can* be done rather than what cannot. However, with a diagnosis of dementia there is a legal responsibility to report the diagnosis to the DVLA, the same as for other medical conditions such as epilepsy or diabetes. If this is not done, then a person could be fined £1,000 and be prosecuted if involved in an accident (DVLA 2023). It is also necessary to inform the insurance company that a diagnosis of dementia has been given – not doing so may render the insurance invalid in the case of an accident, whether or not it was the fault of the person diagnosed with dementia. When the DVLA is informed there are three potential outcomes. The person may be required to undertake a driving assessment, be able to continue driving or be required to surrender their license.

HOW DRIVING ABILITY IS ASSESSED

In the first instance the DVLA will seek medical advice (e.g., GP, MAS specialist) about the person's ability to drive. From this medical advice the DVLA may request the person takes a driving assessment at an assessment centre in the person's area, and this takes between one and two hours (see Dementia UK leaflet in resources). The test will usually consist of an interview, a reaction test and an on-road driving assessment. If the DVLA have requested the assessment, the report will be sent outlining the recommendations from the driving assessment. The decision made will then be communicated by the DVLA to the person with dementia.

It is worth noting that if a person or their carer is concerned about driving and they have not been given advice to stop driving by the GP or memory service, they can arrange a driving assessment privately via a driving mobility centre of which there are about 20 across the UK. The cost will vary depending on if you have self-referred or have been referred by an organization, such as the DVLA (see Driving Mobility website in the Resources section).

CONTINUING TO DRIVE

Over the age of 70 a person must renew their licence every three years. When a person has a diagnosis of dementia, if initially deemed fit to drive, the DVLA will usually issue a new license for a shorter period of time (usually one year), and it will need to be reapplied for at the end of that time period. However, if changes in ability are noticed before the end of that time period, then stopping driving at that point may be necessary.

If a driving assessment has been undertaken, they will have issued guidance about managing risks specific to that person. However, there are practical things that the person should think about, for example driving in daylight wherever possible, when driving alone taking routes that are familiar, avoiding distractions when driving, and avoiding certain types of roads, such as busy motorways.

Whilst a person is still driving it may be helpful to support them to start to consider the future and to actively plan for the time when they are no longer able to drive. The 'driving and dementia decision aid' is a useful tool that may guide a person through this form of planning ahead (see Resources section).

IF A PERSON CAN NO LONGER DRIVE

If the decision is made that a person can no longer drive, they must surrender their licence straight away and stop driving. People should also be aware that if their license is revoked, they can appeal the decision but should not drive whilst the appeal is ongoing. In some instances, a person with dementia may have their licence revoked but will continue to drive. This may be due to several possible reasons: they may not have sufficient insight and believe they can drive safely, they may forget that they are not allowed to drive, or they may refuse to accept the decision of the DVLA and the clinicians.

Family members can find this particularly difficult to manage as they feel a responsibility and know they should do something but have the emotional burden of feeling they are betraying the person they care for (Liddle et al. 2015). If discussing driving cessation with the person with dementia is unsuccessful, contacting their GP and asking their advice as to how to manage this may be useful. A decision will then be made as to who will report the person to the DVLA for the safety of the person with dementia, other road users and pedestrians.

APPROACHING CONVERSATIONS ABOUT DRIVING

As in this case study, discussing stopping driving with someone may be difficult as it can arouse strong feelings. There is not an easy way to have these conversations but here are some suggestions that may help:

- If possible, approach the subject in a collaborative way. Although Albert was unhappy about stopping driving, taking time to talk through the issues, whether a family member or healthcare professional, may result in the person deciding to stop driving voluntarily. This is preferable as being able to make the decision independently helps with their sense of control over the situation, rather than feeling forced into stopping driving.

- Ideally this subject will have already been discussed before attending an appointment to receive a diagnosis, so the person and their family are aware of the potential impact a diagnosis of dementia may have on their ability to drive. It can be hard for a family to take in all the information given at the time when a diagnosis is delivered. It is not unusual for a family affected by dementia to express surprise that *they* should have contacted the DVLA following the diagnosis. There is a lot for them to take in and often emotions are high.

- When advising a family member in how to discuss driving with the person they support, suggest that this is done in a relaxed way, for example, picking a time when the person is more relaxed and receptive about talking about the diagnosis and what it means for them and the family. There may be times of day that are best avoided to raise the issue, such as when the person is tired. When having the conversation keep calm and if they are becoming unhappy move on to another subject rather than letting things escalate, as it will be harder to revisit the discussion if it has ended in conflict. Sometimes having some information to leave with the person with dementia to look at in their own time may be helpful, such as Dementia UK's driving and dementia leaflet (see Resources section).

LIFE WITHOUT A CAR

Giving up driving can be practically and emotionally difficult and thought needs to be given to suggesting alternative forms of transport that support continued independence (Holden and Pusey 2021). Information about local transport schemes, taxi cards and community transport offers can be helpful. The local authority will be able to advise on any local initiatives.

The practicalities of what to do with the car if it is not going to be used any more is something that needs to be approached with sensitivity and the solution will be different for each person. Solutions like giving the car to a family member, maybe a grandchild who has just passed their test, will help the person with dementia feel that they have done something worthwhile with it. Alternatively selling it could help to raise some money that could go towards taxis or other forms of transport.

Some people may wish to keep the car, possibly on the drive so they can continue to care for it and have it available for family members to use to take them to places that they need to go. However, serious consideration needs to be given to this option; for example would it distress the person living with dementia to see it there? Is there a possibility that they could forget they cannot drive, and try to go out in the car? There is also a financial implication as the car would need to be taxed and insured still.

In the case of Albert care would need to be taken to reassure him that not driving should not mean that he cannot do the things he loves such as playing bowls and attending church activities. Maybe friends could offer to give him a lift or it be suggested that some of the money he saves from not driving be put aside specifically for taxis to the places he wants to go. The professional working with them may want to explore whether family could offer to take them shopping, or if they could do an internet shop and have their food delivered.

SUPPORTING POSSIBLE REACTIONS WHEN A PERSON IS NO LONGER ABLE TO DRIVE

A person with dementia and their family may each react in a variety of ways when being told the person is no longer able to drive. These could include anger, denial, relief or fear for the future. Health and social care clinicians need to be sensitive to the potential for a range of reactions and offer emotional support and validation of their feelings (using empathy and active listening to make the person feel heard and understood), alongside practical support. Stopping driving could also cause feelings of grief and loss that should not be underestimated and those supporting should offer the person support in expressing their feelings. It might be helpful to refer the person with dementia and/or their family carer to the Admiral Nurse Dementia Helpline for more specialist support (see Sources of Support section).

CONCLUSION

For a person receiving a diagnosis of dementia, being told not to drive can be traumatic, raising many questions and feelings. Care needs to be taken to ensure that the person has all the relevant information they need and that their emotions are always taken into consideration. Supporting a person and the family throughout this time can take a mix of skills, careful communication and awareness on the part of the supporting professional.

SOURCES OF SUPPORT

If you have any questions about helping a person with any aspect of dementia, call our free Helpline on 0800 888 6678 or email at helpline@dementiauk.org
If you would prefer a pre-booked appointment by phone or video, call via the Dementia UK website: www.dementiauk.org

RESOURCES

Medical conditions, disabilities and driving. www.gov.uk/driving-medical-conditions
Dementia UK. Driving and dementia. www.dementiauk.org/wp-content/uploads/2022/10/Driving-and-dementia.pdf
Older drivers. www.olderdrivers.org.uk/driver-assessment/find-a-driver-assessment
Driving and dementia decision aid. https://adhere.org.au/drivingdementia
Driving mobility. www.drivingmobility.org.uk

REFERENCES

Bennett, J.M. (2022) *Dementia and driving: A cognitive test approach* (Doctoral dissertation, Macquarie University).
Driving and Vehicle Licensing Authority (DVLA) (2023) *Driving and dementia.* www.gov.uk/dementia-and-driving
Holden, A. & Pusey, H. (2021) The impact of driving cessation for people with dementia: An integrative review. *Dementia.* 20(3): 1105–1123.
Liddle, J., Tan, A., Liang, P. et al. (2015) 'The biggest problem we've ever had to face': How families manage driving cessation with people with dementia. *International Psychogeriatrics.* 28(1): 109–122.
Wilson, S. & Pinner, G. (2013) Driving and dementia: A clinician's guide. *Advances in Psychiatric Treatment.* 19(2): 89–96.

CHAPTER 14

Supporting people with dementia at home who are at risk of falling

INTRODUCTION

Falls are a common and often devastating problem amongst older people, with the potential to cause morbidity, mortality and increased use of healthcare services including premature nursing home admissions. A simple accident like slipping on a wet floor can be life changing for an older person and may result in reduced confidence and injury, such as a fracture. For older people, a broken bone can also be the start of more serious health problems and can lead to long-term disability. Most of these falls are associated with one or more identifiable risk factors, such as muscle weakness, an unsteady gait or effects of certain medications. In the advent of services that now target the risk of falling, there has been a reduction in falls and serious injury. People with dementia may have other co-morbid conditions which can increase their risk of falls, and the symptoms of the dementia itself may make someone more at risk of falling. However falls are not an inevitable part of living with dementia, and much can be done to manage the risk. The case study below highlights some of the difficulties faced by health and social care practitioners in assessing and managing falls risk in people with dementia, and following this a dementia specialist nurse (Admiral Nurse) will respond with advice on how to support a person with dementia and their family carer when there is a risk of falling.

Anthony MacKay, Falls Coordinator

From my experience as a falls coordinator, dementia doesn't always happen in isolation, and patients can also experience a wide range of other co-morbidities. These can be age related, such as reduced mobility, poor balance and sight problems, or due to long-term conditions such as chronic obstructive pulmonary disease or diabetes. People with dementia are also at higher risk of falling due to the nature of the condition, whether in hospital or in their own homes.

One family I worked with consisted of a wife who was caring for her husband with dementia who constantly had a need to 'go somewhere'. The challenge was that the husband was quite mobile but unable to process the risks of constantly getting up and walking around day and night. This led to several falls and his wife not getting much sleep due to the constant fear her husband was going to get up during the night and leave the home. Eventually the husband did leave the home and ended up falling and being admitted to hospital.

Falls are multi-factorial and can cause increased stress and anxiety for family carers and may lead them to be risk averse, which in itself can lead to the person with dementia becoming deconditioned due to an imposed reduced mobility. This may also lead to further challenges when trying to keep them safe and trying to gain compliance of the person with dementia with falls-related safety issues. Once someone falls the risk of falling again is increased and can also lead to fear of falling which then can become a self-fulfilling prophecy, as the focus becomes narrowed to the exclusion of other risk factors. People need to lead happy and fulfilling lives and some falls risks may need to be mitigated against but also balanced so as not to unduly restrain a person's freedom.

The environment a person with dementia inhabits, whether that be their own home or a hospital ward, cannot be totally 'risk free' and therefore education around having a prepared plan for a fall, and in the worst case a 'long lie', which is where a person waits on the floor for more than one hour after falling, is recommended. This can also give some control back to patient and carer and reduce the fear and anxiety about 'what if'. Patients and carers need support and being able to access support groups where other people can share their experiences is invaluable.

Kerry Lyons, Consultant Admiral Nurse,
Physical Health and Frailty

DEMENTIA AND FALLS

Within the case study, Anthony refers to a range of challenges when considering how to care for and support a person with dementia and their carer with an increased risk of falling. He also refers to the fact that both near misses and actual falls can lead to a loss of independence, confidence and, where a fall is sustained, distress, pain and injury.

It is important to remember that falling is not an inevitable part of ageing (NICE 2019). Anyone can experience a fall, but as we age, our risk of falling increases. A third of adults over the age of 65 years, and half of people over the age of 80 years, will experience at least one fall per year (Close and Lord 2022). Falls are common in people with dementia, who are two to three times more likely to experience a fall than older people without dementia. Falls can result in serious injury, such as a fracture or head injury. It is important to remember that whilst risk of falling increases with age, people with young onset dementia may also be susceptible to falls due to the symptoms of their dementia. Increased risk of falling in people with dementia is associated with the following factors identified in Box 14.1.

Box 14.1: Factors associated with falls in older people

→ impaired judgment

→ altered visual impairment

→ altered sensory perception

→ decreasing mobility amidst increasing frailty and sarcopenia (progressive and generalized loss of skeletal muscle mass and strength)

→ poor balance and coordination

→ increasing confusion and disorientation which creates difficulties in communicating and expressing need

---

→ polypharmacy.

(NICE 2019)

The majority of falls and fractures in older people can be prevented, and as Anthony points out, the most valuable intervention is to recognize and assess the risk and likelihood of a person falling, alongside identifying and treating the wide range of underlying factors which may contribute to that risk (see Box 14.1).

FALLS RISK: DEMENTIA AND OTHER CO-MORBID CONDITIONS

Dementia is often experienced by an individual alongside other co-morbid conditions. For example, when frailty is co-morbid with dementia the impact of emerging and increasing frailty can be overshadowed by dementia, especially if we focus all our caring interventions on one 'primary' condition, and the associated symptoms. This is called diagnostic overshadowing. Diagnostic overshadowing can also mean that dementia is seen as the primary and causative factor for a fall and detract from considering other conditions.

For example, bone fragility, such as in osteoporosis, is also a risk factor for falls and injury, and should be incorporated into a falls risk assessment. Fragility fractures more commonly occur in hips, wrists and the spine, with hip fractures accounting for around 1.8 million hospital bed days each year (OHID 2022). Knowing a person's medical history and co-morbid conditions, such as osteoporosis with low mineral bone density, will help us to understand if the person has an increased risk of sustaining a fragility fracture from low-level, low-energy falls (falls which usually would not result in a severe injury) (Dautzenberg et al. 2021).

Other risk factors are low weight (BMI<19), poor diet lacking in vitamin D and calcium, diabetes, alcohol, smoking and long-term drug therapy, such as corticosteroids (see NICE guideline in the Resources section).

EARLY CONSIDERATIONS FOR PRACTICE

As a professional, an excellent starting point to improving falls management within dementia care is to routinely consider the areas listed in Table 14.1 within your assessment(s).

Table 14.1: Considerations in assessments (Gillespie et al. 2012)

History of falls.	Identify potential risks in the person's environment.
Complete a risk assessment tool.	Take a detailed history of where falls have taken place, identifying what happened, where and what time of the day.
Assess the level of frailty.	Use a frailty index or measurement tool and consider multi-professional involvement and onward referral to specialist services.
Observe for anomalies in mobility, balance and gait.	If any observed it is important to explore the underlying cause(s) and, where necessary, make an onward referral to specialist services.
Assess for pain.	Use a validated pain assessment tool if pain is considered a causative factor in a fall.
Assess level of understanding of dementia.	Ascertain the family's knowledge and understanding of dementia and the impact this might have on a risk of falling.
Assess medication effects in relation to drowsiness, unsteadiness and falls.	Review all prescribed medications as some may carry a risk of falls as a side-effect and consider possible medication interactions.
Assess for other medical conditions increasing the risk of falls, e.g., diabetes.	Advise and guide on the importance of healthy ageing and promote the importance of attending monitoring appointments and annual health reviews.
Emotional support for the person with dementia and their family.	Offer reassurance to the person with dementia and their family throughout the process, and advise what to do after a fall.

Finding the root cause

Once you have considered all the above, a good starting point in finding out the root cause of falls is to refer a person to their GP. The person's GP will be able to undertake or initiate a range of tests and investigations to ascertain a potential cause(s) for an identified falls risk (Bruce et al. 2021). If the person is also identified as being frail, this assessment may be captured as part of a comprehensive geriatric assessment.

OTHER SERVICES AND WHAT CAN BE OFFERED

There are a range of services, interventions and support that can reduce the risk of falls (Table 14.2).

Table 14.2: Services, interventions and support for falls prevention

Services	Interventions and support
General practitioner	• Electrocardiogram to exclude bradycardia, asystole and tachycardia • Checking for blood pressure problems • Referral for ophthalmology review • Referral to audiology • Assessment of bone health and possible DEXA scan to check bone density • Medication review • Pain assessment • Referral to specialist falls prevention service
Specialist falls prevention service	• Investigating the root cause of the person's falls • Identification and management of risks • Promotion of independence • Improving the person's postural stability • Providing healthy living advice • Improving mobility confidence and reducing fear of falling
Physiotherapy	• Assessing the person's falls risk and advising on activities and interventions to reduce this • Offering guidance and strategies for safe movement • Guidance on mobility aids • Assessing a person's suitability for engagement in a strength and balance training programme
Occupational therapist	• Identifying daily activities that a person may find difficult and offering practical ways to modify tasks, support care interventions and aid independence • Offering assessment and advice on home equipment and adaptations

Both physiotherapists and occupational therapists offer advice on everyday issues, such as getting in and out of a car, moving around the home and navigating tight or difficult spaces in the home. Such advice and guidance is useful to the person with dementia but can also offer solutions for a family carer in enabling them to care in the safest way. It is not uncommon for a person who is at risk of falling to lose independence and become increasingly isolated due to not wanting to leave their home. This is also the case for people with dementia. As Anthony states, in some cases, this inactivity can compound the situation through clinical deconditioning. Promoting wellness, pursuing the least restrictive options, and enabling independence and confidence are important aspects when advising families on how to live as well as possible with dementia. Anthony talked about the anxiety experienced by carers amidst an escalating falls risk; it is important to actively listen and act on their concerns to make a positive impact.

ENVIRONMENTAL INTERVENTIONS

Many falls happen in the home; however, hazards in the home can be either managed or mitigated. As professionals, we have an opportunity to see a person's home environment with 'fresh eyes' in terms of falls risk, and in doing so we can advise on small changes that improve both safety and independence.

There are adaptations and small changes that can reduce a person's risk of falls within the home. Suggest to the person and their family that decluttering outside spaces, and ensuring pathways are even, clear and well-lit, can significantly reduce the risk of falls. Installation of carefully placed grab rails or converting steps into a ramp can be helpful. When the person with dementia leaves the house ensure they use appropriate, prescribed walking aids and that they are maintained and remain in good condition and working order.

Correctly fitting footwear with a sturdy sole and good grip can prevent some falls; this may mean moving to a lace-up or Velcro shoe fastening for a more secure fit. Advice can also be offered on 'when' to go out, as falls are more likely to occur when pavements are wet or icy, and visibility is poor, or when the person is more tired, unsteady and less alert.

Inside the home

The person with dementia and their family could be advised to keep entrances and hallways clear, so it is easy to get in and out of the property, removing unnecessary rugs or ensuring that their edges are secure (products are available at most flooring outlets). All floors should be kept clear of clutter and any trailing wires or cables should be removed or secured. Essential objects such as spectacles and remote controls should be easily reached, to prevent overstretching and overbalancing.

A person with dementia can be at risk of falling when unsure of their way around the home so using visual cues, prompts and reminders will help both orientation and wayfinding. Bannisters and securely fitted stair carpets can reduce a falls risk. Any furniture with thin legs could be tripped over or may collapse if the person leans or bumps into them.

Modifying the bathroom environment can not only reduce a falls risk, but also improve a person's continence. Fitting a toilet seat that is a contrasting colour from the toilet makes it easy to see and keeping the toilet seat up enables the person to sit quickly and easily. Using coloured toilet paper on a freestanding holder ensures that it is easy to see and within reach. Using non-slip mats on the bathroom floor, in the bath, and in the shower, alongside removing trip hazards such as toilet and pedestal sink rugs can help to prevent trips and falls.

Good lighting throughout the home is essential, and high wattage light bulbs should be advised for the main house lights. A landing, night or movement sensitive light can be useful to ensure the person who gets up in the night can see where to go and avoid hazards. The installation of grab rails at useful points will also enable a safer route to the bathroom during the night. An occupational therapy assessment could introduce a shower chair, bath seat, toilet frame and/or raised toilet seat, to aid independence and reduce a risk of falls. There are also a range of independent living equipment and assistive technologies that could reduce the risk of night-time falls, for example movement sensors and fall detectors (see Resources section).

MISPERCEPTIONS AND VISUAL PROBLEMS

Visual difficulties in dementia can create misperceptions and illusions that can lead to increased confusion, anxiety, distress and falls, so good lighting is essential, and shadows should be minimized. More natural light can be achieved in the home by fitting light, coloured curtains in the living room and removing net curtains or blinds (though using a blackout variety in the bedroom will aid sleep). Patterned carpets, curtains and rugs may cause confusion for a person with dementia, as they may misinterpret patterns as gradients, steps or uneven surfaces. They may also struggle to separate objects and backgrounds of similar colours (Bruce et al. 2021). Block colours are better in reducing misperceptions, rather than busy patterned carpets or wallpaper.

However, it may not be possible to change the home environment for many reasons, not least the cost of doing so may be prohibitive. If changes are considered, then advising a matt finish for flooring and walls is preferable as gloss surfaces may appear slippery or wet and cause fear and uncertainty for a person with dementia when mobilizing. If flooring is being changed then using one colour/type of carpet or flooring throughout the property will reduce falls that occur when moving from one surface to another, for example from carpet to vinyl flooring.

A different colour between walls and flooring will give contrast and aid distinguishing the edges of the room. Similarly, brighter and stronger colours may be easier to distinguish than pastels. Distinguishing the top and bottom steps in a staircase with strips, and outlining door frames, plug sockets or light switches, painting them or marking them out using tape in a contrasting shade or colour, may help the person with dementia to see them better.

Additionally, advice may be given on removing or covering mirrors when they are not in use, as this can contribute to falls risk if the person is struggling to see and identify themselves within the reflection.

THE IMPORTANCE OF SLEEP

Poor-quality sleep can negatively impact both the person with dementia and their carer. Many people with dementia become increasingly confused and unsteady at night, making falls more likely. People with dementia can experience a range of changes in their circadian rhythm, so it is not uncommon to experience excessive sleeping during daytime hours and a disturbed night-time sleep pattern. Poor sleep can also lead to carer exhaustion and burnout as identified by Anthony in his case study.

Advising on good sleep hygiene

Sleep disturbance can increase the risk of falls. There is advice you can offer to promote good sleep, such as:

- Avoid stimulants, such as caffeine, nicotine and alcohol.

- Review medication effects on sleep quality.

- Identify and treat underlying sleep disorders and pain.

- Identify and manage any issues around nocturia.

- Ensure the bedroom environment promotes sleep (see section above on Environmental Interventions).

- Promote good day and night-time routines, such as limiting daytime naps and increasing natural daylight exposure.

- Encourage physical activity and regular exercise to tolerance.

- Encourage social activity and meaningful engagement through the day.

Medication options to aid sleep in dementia should be used as a last resort and considered after all other interventions have been thoroughly explored. Such sedation must be carefully balanced against the risk of increased confusion and falls.

BEING PREPARED IN CASE OF A FALL

As Anthony stated, as well as advising on risk prevention and reduction, professionals can offer education on what to do should a fall occur. It is important to be prepared for the possibility of falls. It may also be helpful to refer a person for a personal alarm, such as telecare, worn in pendant form or on the wrist that can be either activated by pressing the unit, or by the internal sensor detecting a fall from a height.

You may advise careful placement of items such as phone handsets, warm blankets and bottles of water in case the person falls whilst on their own and cannot get up from the floor. Devices such as Alexa™, Siri™ or other voice-activated systems can be useful to call a family member, neighbour or emergency service in the case of a fall when the person cannot get up.

The person with dementia and their family could also be advised to think how emergency services and support can access their property should the person fall. A key safe with a code to allow people to access the key, nominating a trusted keyholder and placing next of kin contact information in a prominent position within the property (e.g., a hallway table) can be helpful.

NEAR MISSES

The family carer should be advised that if a person with dementia begins to fall from an upright position, they should not attempt to catch them or stop their fall. Instead, they should try to control their fall by lowering them to the floor. Advise the carer to seek urgent support even if it is a near miss and a fall does not occur, as these are often vital opportunities to put in place additional preventative measures to reduce the risk of future falls. It also offers an opportunity to support the person and their carer, as falls can be a distressing occurrence.

WHAT TO DO IF A FALL HAPPENS

It is important for everyone to keep calm when a fall occurs. There may be benefit in you walking through strategies with the family on how to deal with a fall, including:

Falls without apparent injury

1. Assess for injuries first; if there are no injuries and it is safe for the person to get up, support them to do so slowly and steadily.

2. Call on a family member, friend or neighbour if needed to help you get the person up safely.

3. To get the person up, ask them to roll onto their hands and knees; using a stable item of furniture such as a heavy chair for support, ask the person to hold onto this item with both hands and rise slowly until upright.

4. Once the person is upright, ask them to sit down and rest.

Falls when injury is suspected, or the person cannot get up safely

1. If you suspect that the person is hurt, or if they are unable to get up, then you should call for immediate help. If the person wears a personal alarm, they should activate this; otherwise, ring 999.

2. If the person has a more minor injury or you think they should be checked over, they should request an urgent appointment with their GP.

3. If there is a warm blanket to hand, you should cover the person's legs until help arrives.

Keep the person comfortable, and if it is possible/safe to do so, try to change their position slightly every 30 minutes to reduce the risk of pressure damage to the skin.

Post-fall assessment

It is important to undertake a post-fall assessment including a review of their falls plan and developing a new and emerging falls risk(s) plan. When a fall occurs, a critical aspect of aftercare should be that a re-assessment is undertaken to re-evaluate any falls management plans in place, identify underlying contributory factors, and take appropriate timely action.

CONCLUSION

Although falls are a common occurrence in people with dementia, not everyone with the diagnosis will experience a fall. Most falls often result in a minor injury, but those which result in a serious injury can often lead to a significant shift in confidence, functional baseline and overall ability to live independently. There are a wide range of actions that we can consider when caring for a person with dementia who is experiencing increasing falls risk, and in supporting their family carer. As Anthony stated, it is important to recognize that falls are often multi-factorial in terms of causation; therefore, we should be considering a wide range of approaches to identifying, mitigating and managing falls risk for families with dementia.

SOURCES OF SUPPORT

If you have any questions about helping a person with any aspect of dementia, call our free Helpline on 0800 888 6678 or email at helpline@dementiauk.org
If you would prefer a pre-booked appointment by phone or video, call via the Dementia UK website: www.dementiauk.org

RESOURCES

Independent Age. Technology to help you at home. https://www.indepen dentage.org/get-advice/health-and-care/help-at-home/technology-to-keep-you-safe-at-home
Comprehensive geriatric assessment. www.bgs.org.uk/cgatoolkit
NICE. Falls in older people: assessing risk and prevention. Clinical guideline [CG161]. www.nice.org.uk/guidance/cg161/chapter/1-recommendations

REFERENCES

Bruce, J., Hossain, A., Lall, R. et al. (2021) Fall prevention interventions in primary care to reduce fractures and falls in people aged 70 years and over: The PreFIT three-arm cluster RCT. *Health Technology Assessment.* 25: 1–114.

Close, J.C.T. & Lord, S.R. (2022) Fall prevention in older people: Past, present and future. *Age & Ageing.* 51(6): afac105. https://doi:10.1093/ageing/afac105

Dautzenberg, L., Beglinger, S., Tsokani, S. et al. (2021) Interventions for preventing falls and fall-related fractures in community-dwelling older adults: A systematic review and network meta-analysis. *JAGS.* 69: 2973–2984.

Gillespie, L.D., Robertson, M.C., Gillespie, W.J. et al. (2012) Interventions for preventing falls in older people living in the community. *Cochrane Database Systematic Reviews.* 2012(9): CD007146. https://doi:10.1002/14651858.CD007146.pub3

National Institute for Health and Care Excellence (NICE) (2019) *Surveillance of falls in older people: Assessing risk and prevention (Guideline CG161).* www.nice.org.uk/guidance/cg161/resources/2019-surveillance-of-falls-in-older-people-assessing-risk-and-prevention-nice-guideline-cg161-pdf-8792148103909

Office for Health Improvement and Disparities (OHID) (2022) *Falls: Applying All Our Health.* www.gov.uk/government/publications/falls-applying-all-our-health/falls-applying-all-our-health

CHAPTER 15

Dementia care when the family carer is frail

INTRODUCTION

There is a growing literature on frailty in people with dementia. However, often overlooked is the impact that frailty can have on an older carer, in terms of their own wellbeing and their ability to meet the care needs of the person with dementia. We know that frailty increases with age and affects almost half of those over the age of 65 (Fogg et al. 2022), so recognizing frailty in older carers of people with dementia is paramount to supporting the whole family.

There is some evidence that being an older carer can increase their risk of experiencing frailty (Potier et al. 2018), and as the case study below demonstrates, frailty in an older carer can negatively impact their mental and physical health, as well as potentially putting the person with dementia at risk of unintentional neglect.

The following case study highlights the difficulties associated with supporting an older couple affected by dementia where the wife, and main carer, is also experiencing frailty. Following this a dementia specialist nurse (Admiral Nurse) advises professionals what they can do if they suspect frailty in an older carer of someone with dementia, and what support can be offered.

Sophie Wellman, General Practitioner

A few years ago, I worked with a couple called Jim and Isla White. I initially visited as Isla had been diagnosed with diabetes and I was there as her GP to discuss this and check some things with her. Isla also struggled with her mobility due to extensive osteoarthritis. She used a stick to mobilize around the house but even with this her balance was not very good and she was assessed as being at risk of falling. Whilst there I became aware of Jim, her husband, who had Alzheimer's disease. During my initial visit to the couple my focus was on Isla and the management of her diabetes, and therefore I did not interact with Jim initially.

However, on my second visit, I was called to see Jim specifically as there was some concern regarding his legs, which were swollen. Whilst there I could see his mobility was very poor and he could only mobilize a couple of steps with his frame. I also observed that his clothes were quite dirty and stained. When he was trying to mobilize, Isla was talking to him in quite a stern domineering manner and trying to almost force him to be mobile. My concerns for each of them increased. I asked about the family and discovered there was a son that lived abroad but no one locally who could help them. I asked how they got their food, and they said that a neighbour did some shopping for them. I then asked if I could check in their fridge and found there was not much food there at all, just some tomatoes and milk.

With the couple's consent I referred them to social services, as I was concerned that they needed much more support to stay independent at home. They seemed happy with this as they felt that they would get support with shopping and keeping the house clean.

Carers were subsequently put in place and the couple were better supported. Unfortunately, Isla became more and more hostile towards the carers whenever they tried to help Jim. She would argue that he didn't need help with washing and other care tasks. The carers contacted us at the GP surgery as they noticed that the house was now smelling of urine. I visited again and realized that both Jim and Isla were sleeping downstairs, one on the sofa and one in a chair. They often could not make it to the upstairs toilet, hence the smell of urine. Isla's mobility had decreased, and I could see that she really struggled to help Jim at all. I tried to discuss the need for increased care but Isla's pride and her denial of the fact that they were struggling made this very difficult, and so she was resistant to all my suggestions. Jim lacked capacity to make any decisions regarding his future care and on the surface would just agree with Isla and had no understanding of the implications of his agreement with Isla. The social work team were equally concerned about the couple's situation.

Unfortunately, a few weeks later Isla went on to have a stroke and was admitted to hospital. This changed things as Jim could not stay safely in the home on his own and was moved into emergency residential care.

Jim and Isla's story highlights the impact that frailty in an older carer can have on their ability to care, and the outcomes for the person with dementia. I often reflect upon this case as I feel that it would have been much better for the couple to have had time to plan for their future care needs. It is sad that decisions had to be made for them in a crisis situation rather than them having input into their future care decisions. I would have liked to have had more conversations with Isla about her own care needs, as looking after Jim put a huge pressure on her physically and mentally.

Kerry Lyons, Consultant Admiral Nurse
for Physical Health and Frailty

OVERVIEW OF FRAILTY AND HOW IT IS ASSESSED

Frailty is a common condition that occurs in around 50% of people over the age of 85 (Gale et al. 2015) and is often framed as a person's inability to 'bounce back' from what can be a relatively minor injury or illness. Frailty is a state of health, which can be referred to as a long-term condition or syndrome. It relates to a person's physical and mental resilience; some refer to this as 'slowing down', however, as with Isla's case, a person may not be initially diagnosed with or recognize themselves as frail. This lack of recognition and inability to forward-plan for current and future care needs can often place a couple, such as Isla and Jim, in increasingly vulnerable clinical and social situations.

As frailty increases, a person steadily becomes more and more vulnerable to minor changes in their personal circumstances, and this vulnerability can have an increasingly negative impact on their health, wellbeing, independence and ability to care for themselves and others. In such cases, being able to identify and then manage a person's frailty can have a significant and positive effect on influencing their health and social care outcomes, alongside preventing potential crisis situations that could lead to unnecessary and lengthy hospital stays, which often lead to poorer clinical outcomes (Hoogendijk et al. 2019).

STAGES OF FRAILTY

There are three stages of frailty: mild, moderate and severe. However, it is important to note that a person's degree of frailty is not always static and may be made better with the right intervention, care and support. The physical characteristics of frailty are weight loss, poor nutrition, hydration issues, fatigue, weakness, reduced physical activity and general 'slowing down' (Xue 2011). Being able to assess and identify frailty will aid supportive interventions that help to manage the person's symptoms over the trajectory of the condition.

There are key markers within the case study indicating Isla's advancing frailty:

- advancing age with evident slowing down

- co-morbidity

- increasing immobility due to extensive osteoarthritis (sleeping downstairs with issues climbing the stairs)

- sarcopenia (reduced muscle mass) creating diminishing strength and balance which contributed to an increasing risk for falls

- suspected urinary incontinence

- increasing inability to care for 'self', and unintentional neglect of others in their care (in this case, Jim).

In the case study Sophie reports that on her second visit to the couple she was specifically called to review Jim; through her description, we can also see key markers of his advancing frailty:

- advancing age with evident slowing down

- co-morbidity

- advancing Alzheimer's disease with associated needs (reliance on Isla for all care needs and decision making)
- increasing immobility (described as only mobile for short distances with a walking frame)
- sleeping downstairs with issues climbing the stairs, indicating diminishing muscle mass, strength and balance
- suspected urinary incontinence
- self-neglect due to inability to care for self.

As in Jim's case, it is not uncommon for a person living with other long-term conditions to also have frailty; however, this may be overlooked by a professional if the focus of care is purely on their main condition such as Alzheimer's disease. To prevent this form of diagnostic overshadowing, it is important to recognize that frailty might not be apparent, unless we actively consider the possibility through formal assessment (Rahman 2019).

UNDERSTANDING FRAILTY SYNDROME

There are five elements to frailty syndrome, and the presence of one or more of these should raise a suspicion that a person may also be living with overall frailty. These elements are falls, immobility, delirium, incontinence and susceptibility to side effects of medication. We note in the case study that both Isla and Jim individually experienced at least two of these elements. Preventing and/or managing elements that contribute to frailty is important when managing the risks associated with emerging and increasing frailty.

SUPPORTING BOTH PARTIES

Dementia is characterized by a progressive deterioration of a person's cognition, and in Jim's case left him with increasing difficulty in performing his activities of daily living. The impact of this often leads to higher levels of dependency and disability, which can have a significant and negative effect on the emotional, psychological and physical wellbeing of carers; especially if added to their caring role they face their own increasing healthcare challenges (Sandilyan and Dening 2019).

IDENTIFYING EMERGING NEEDS AND ACCEPTING SUPPORT

Supporting a carer to adapt to change, especially amidst the need at times to step back from their physical caring role, can be a challenging situation to navigate. However, there are several things we can do to support a carer to still feel involved in care and decision making, which may make it easier for them to accept outside care and support. When a carer refuses outside help, it is important to try to understand the underlying reasons; there may be a combination of reasons affecting their decision to refuse support, such as fear of loss of role, or any of the following:

- fear of others thinking they aren't coping

- failure to carry out their 'duty' and worry that people may think they don't care for the person with dementia

- previous experience of poor care or support

- fear of loss of role and purpose

- worry that accepting help may leave them vulnerable

- loss of control over their lives and situation

- worry what other family members may think about them accepting care and support

- cost of care and support.

Establishing what their fears or concerns are and then talking them through can help the person come to terms with accepting support. It also enables conversations that lead to their understanding of the outcome of accepting care that can enable them to live safely and longer in their own home. For many families affected by dementia this is often an overarching desire and symbolic for them of their independence and autonomy.

Caring for someone with dementia, whilst also living with their own increasing frailty, can be challenging, but understanding more about the level of emerging frailty and associated needs can be an excellent first step to them seeking the right care and support.

HOW WILL A PERSON BE ASSESSED FOR FRAILTY?

There are a range of frailty screening and assessment tools currently used by healthcare practitioners (which one to use is often decided through local guidance and policy). Most are referred to as Clinical Frailty Scores or Clinical Frailty Scales. In simple terms, all that a tool will do is identify a degree of fitness and frailty to classify the stage into one of the three main categories: mild, moderate, and severe (see Table 15.1).

Table 15.1: The three stages of frailty

Mild	Person may appear to be 'slowing down', increasingly needing help with everyday tasks, such as meal preparation, finance planning, heavy housework, medication management and transportation. They may also have an unsteady gait and be unable to walk alone outside. Typically, they may walk with a frame.
Moderate	Person will need help with all outside activities, alongside needing support with all elements of housekeeping. They will often have problems with the use of stairs and will require some assistance to bathe and dress (this assistance may be prompting, guidance or just supervision).
Severe	Person will be dependent on carer support, and therefore require full assistance with all aspects of care needs.

NEXT STEPS AFTER FRAILTY ASSESSMENT

If you suspect a person has undiagnosed frailty, as a health or social care professional you are ideally placed to refer the person for a frailty assessment, or you may undertake the screening yourself, if able to do this as part of your role. One of the most important things we can all do as professionals is use the opportunity our personal contact affords to discuss the possibility of frailty and to either signpost or, with consent, make a referral to the appropriate services. This ensures a family can take appropriate next steps in assessment, management and future care planning.

If a person is identified as frail from an initial screening, they should then receive a full assessment of their needs, and this is often referred to as a comprehensive geriatric assessment (CGA). The CGA places the person and their family central to the assessment process based upon their individual needs (Devons 2002), such as any current symptoms and underlying medical conditions. CGA is usually undertaken by a person or a team with expertise in the care and management of frailty and encompasses functional capacity, falls risk, cognition, mood, medication, social support, finances, goals of care and advance care preferences.

In Isla and Jim's case, their frailty assessment would be conducted separately, but the CGA would consider all their needs (both apart and together), alongside acknowledging any current and emerging issues around Isla's primary carer role in supporting Jim with his dementia care.

Table 15.2 shows the several domains of a CGA, and provides areas you might consider in your own assessment.

Table 15.2: Domains of the CGA and areas to consider

Domain	Areas to consider
Functional capacity	Including: mobility, communication, ability to self-care and care for others, self-direction, working tolerance or work skills
Falls risk	Including: current level of falls risk, history of falls and 'near misses', risk of sustaining a fall when caregiving, ability to communicate around actions on movement, identification of factors contributing to increased falls risk and whether these can be mitigated, modified or managed
Cognition	Including: capacity for decision making, level of confusion and orientation, diagnosis, stage and understanding of dementia, stage of any other illness, behaviours and psychological symptoms, delirium history
Mood	Including: issues and/or concerns affecting emotional and psychological wellbeing, and effect of the current situation on relationships, roles and duty when considering co-dependent caregiving situations
Polypharmacy	Including: medication review, deprescribing opportunities, concerns regarding medication administration

Social support and living situation	Including: caring roles/responsibilities (is more help needed?), effect on relationships, roles and duty when considering co-dependent caregiving situations, suitability of the living situation, risk assessment, identify whether care, support, equipment or assistive technology is needed
Financial concerns	Benefit eligibility; identify any other financial concerns
Goals of care and advanced care preferences	Including: insight and understanding of the person(s) living with frailty health and wellbeing, wishes around goals of care and what is realistically achievable, escalation and not for escalation plans (who to reach out to and when), planning for future needs
Nutrition and weight	Including: nutritional and fluid intake, changes in eating or drinking habits, changes in taste, swallowing difficulties, weight change, eating practices, access and ability to plan, purchase and prepare food
Continence	Including: concerns around incontinence and type of continence, routines and times of any issues, falls risk, self-care and self-direction alongside level of care and support needs, urinary tract infection history, genitourinary issues, communication and challenges regarding continence management, products or aids used
Sexual function	Any changes to sexual activity or function as a result of frailty and impact of this on mood
Vision and hearing	Glasses/hearing aids prescribed and if used
Dentition	Oral health and denture use
Spiritual needs	Consider the person's spiritual, religious or cultural needs and wishes

Onward referrals should be considered where indicated, and depending on the identified issue, such as to their GP, a frailty specialist, occupational therapist, physiotherapist, Admiral Nurse, falls prevention team, mental health team, carer support networks, speech and language team, social services, pharmacist, local voluntary services, Citizens Advice, palliative care team, dietician, continence team, optician, audiology, dentist and faith groups.

SUPPORTING FAMILIES TO PLAN

Once the care and support plan is formulated, a response to a CGA can focus on maintaining and optimizing the health and functionality of the person(s) living with frailty alongside consideration of the needs of their carer. A plan should also include a contingency plan of what to do if the person with frailty becomes unwell and who to approach for advice and support. In the case above the contingency planning would focus on both Jim and Isla, but especially for Isla given her role in caring for her spouse with dementia.

CONCLUSION

Dementia and frailty often come together, both in the person with the diagnosis of dementia but also in their older, spousal carers. Frailty can often be unidentified and overshadowed when faced with other conditions, such as dementia. This may lead to families affected by dementia and frailty missing vital opportunities to receive the right support at the right time. By taking the opportunity to screen for frailty, health and social care professionals are well placed to encourage follow up with a comprehensive assessment of needs, such as offered in the CGA, so providing opportunity to plan for both current and future needs. Through such planning supportive conversations can be explored to help address any fears, reduce barriers to accepting care, and help a person and their carer to stay independent for as long as possible.

SOURCES OF SUPPORT

If you have any questions about helping a person with any aspect of dementia, call our free Helpline on 0800 888 6678 or email at helpline@dementiauk.org
If you would prefer a pre-booked appointment by phone or video, call via the Dementia UK website: www.dementiauk.org

RESOURCES

NHS England. Frailty toolkit. www.england.nhs.uk/rightcare/toolkits/frailty
British Geriatrics Society (BGS). Comprehensive geriatric assessment toolkit for primary care practitioners. www.bgs.org.uk/resources/resource-series/comprehensive-geriatric-assessment-toolkit-for-primary-care-practitioners

British Geriatrics Society (BGS). **Joining the dots: A blueprint for preventing and managing frailty in older people.** www.bgs.org.uk/policy-and-media/joining-the-dots-a-blueprint-for-preventing-and-managing-frailty-in-older-people

REFERENCES

Devons, C.A.J. (2002) Comprehensive geriatric assessment: Making the most of the aging years. *Current Opinion Clinical Nutrition and Metabolic Care.* 5: 19–24.

Fogg, C., Fraser, S.D.S., Roderick, P. et al. (2022) The dynamics of frailty development and progression in older adults in primary care in England (2006–2017): A retrospective cohort profile. *BMC Geriatrics.* 22(30). https://doi.org/10.1186/s12877-021-02684-y

Gale, C.R., Cooper, C. & Sayer, A.A. (2015) Prevalence of frailty and disability: Findings from the English Longitudinal Study of Ageing. *Age and Ageing.* 44(1): 162–165.

Hoogendijk, E.O., Afilalo, J., Ensrud, K.E. et al. (2019) Frailty: Implications for clinical practice and public health. *Lancet.* 394(10206): 1365–1375.

Potier, F., Degryse, J.M., Aubouy, G. et al. (2018) Spousal caregiving is associated with an increased risk of frailty: A case-control study. *Journal of Frailty and Aging.* 7(3): 170–175.

Rahman, S. (2019) Frailty: From awareness to identity. In: *Living with frailty: From assets to deficits to resilience.* London: Routledge.

Sandilyan, M.B. & Dening, T. (2019) What is dementia? In: K. Harrison Dening (Ed.), *Evidence-based practice in dementia for nurses and nursing students.* London: Jessica Kingsley Publishers.

Xue, Q.L. (2011) The frailty syndrome: Definition and natural history. *Clinical Geriatric Medicine.* 27(1): 1–15.

CHAPTER 16

Is there a time when it is too late?

ADVANCE CARE PLANNING IN DEMENTIA

INTRODUCTION

There has been a lot of work over the past 15 years to help people in the UK to talk and think more openly about dying, death and bereavement, and to make their own end-of-life plans. Advance care planning (ACP) differs from general care planning in that it is usually used in the context of progressive illness and anticipated deterioration.

The case study below provides an example of how a plan developed to support a person's future care, such as an advance care plan, may have been useful at a critical point in their life. Shiny, a dementia nurse within an acute hospital, describes how she met Magda who had been admitted to an acute hospital for pneumonia. Shiny tried to support the family to start to plan for Magda's future care and her wishes and priorities for such care. Magda was readmitted to the acute hospital with another chest infection and Shiny found that no progress had been made in planning for end of life and care in the form of ACP, so an opportunity was lost for Magda in considering what she wanted for her future care.

Following the case study, a dementia specialist nurse (Admiral Nurse) writes about ACP and what this may include and entail. The Admiral Nurse also offers guidance on how to facilitate and support ACP for a person with dementia and suggests various approaches and resources.

It is essential that health and social care professionals support people with dementia to plan for their future and in making decisions about care and treatment for a time when they lack the ability to do so. It is an important part of exercising autonomy and control over our lives and is considered an essential element in maintaining personhood.

Shiny Varghese, Dementia Nurse in Acute Care

I was on one of our hospital wards reviewing the care needs of Magda, a person with dementia, who had been admitted for a chest infection and was now recovered. Plans were being made for her discharge. Magda's son, Oskar, arrived for a visit so I included him in the review. During my conversation, I asked if Magda had a Lasting Power of Attorney (LPA) for health and welfare, as well as for finance. Oskar responded for his mother and stated that he had not yet got around to this and wanted some clarification about what it entailed. I gave them some verbal information and also provided some written information about LPAs, as well as how to make an advance care plan and an advance decision to refuse treatment, if this was something they might also want to consider. Magda was subsequently discharged from hospital.

I saw Magda again several months later when she was readmitted to the acute hospital for another chest infection. As part of my role as the hospital's dementia nurse, I went to the ward to review Magda's care needs. Oskar was also present in the room and informed me that his mother had deteriorated a lot since the last admission, and he worried that this was his fault and he had not cared for his mother well enough. I tried to reassure Oskar and explained to him that dementia was a progressive disease and about the stages of dementia. I again asked if they had managed to arrange the LPA for health and welfare or had made any advance decisions about what care Magda might or might not want. The son replied that he had not understood the relevance of developing an LPA or advance care plan at that time. Reflecting on our conversations today Oskar now realized the importance of such plans for his mother's care going forward. However, Magda no longer had the capacity to fully participate in and contribute to such planning.

On reflection, I wondered if I had done enough six months ago to promote their engagement in planning ahead. However, it is not straightforward as many other health and social care professionals were involved in Magda's care and at different times, who all could have influenced her to think about her future wishes and preferences for care.

Dio Giotas, Admiral Nurse

WHY IS ADVANCE CARE PLANNING IMPORTANT FOR PEOPLE WITH DEMENTIA?

Dementia is a neurological disorder characterized by a progressive decline in cognitive function and the ability to perform daily activities. Dementia is the leading cause of death in the UK, and it is estimated that by 2040, 220,000 people with dementia will die each year in England and Wales (ONS 2020). People with dementia will often have one or more other long-term conditions which could increase their vulnerability, frailty and the need for an effective and coordinated plan of care.

Deterioration within the context of dementia is often synonymous with palliative care and end of life as the condition progresses with time. Therefore, dementia should be managed as a long-term condition in primary care, along with any other co-morbidities (e.g., diabetes or hypertension) which should also include ACP discussions. Regular health checks (NHS 2020) with the GP or the practice nurse may include bloods tests, medication reviews and referrals to specialists. Signposting to local and national services are required for both the person with dementia and those caring for them and are now expected to include having the opportunity to discuss and plan for future care (NICE 2018).

ACP is seen as being synonymous with the provision of high-quality care and should be accessible to a person with dementia from the point of diagnosis to the end of their life. If ACP is initiated as early as possible after diagnosis it allows time for the person with dementia and their family to fully understand its importance and consider their wishes and preferences for future care. However, as highlighted in Shiny's case study, recognizing the right time and utilizing every opportunity to discuss ACP are key to its implementation.

Planning for the future when diagnosed with a progressive,

long-term condition such as dementia is often a battle against time, especially where capacity to make future care decisions may be lost early in the course of the condition. Such planning can be a lengthy and fragmented process, involving several people, including the person with the diagnosis, family members, carers and supporters and professionals from health and social care settings. However, ACP is an essential component of proactive and person-centred care that everyone should expect to receive as they approach the end stages of their lives.

ACP promotes personhood, agency and authentic participation of the person living with the condition, which are key concepts in modern dementia care. It reduces anxiety about future care dilemmas faced by people with dementia and their families – as health and wellbeing become more fragile, raising the prospect of more frequent or invasive medical interventions (Detering et al. 2010; DH 2008). Done well, ACP is personalized, inclusive and specific to each person, representing their true wishes whilst they still have the mental capacity to communicate them reliably. It is about seeing the person behind the condition, a person that comes from a specific cultural background and can be a way to celebrate that unique identity – reflecting the aspects of ethnicity and culture to be observed, respected and preserved. ACP can also act as a care passport that is shared across community and emergency care services. Ultimately, it reduces repetitions and irons out contradictions between one health or social care setting and another.

WHO CAN INFLUENCE ACP FOR A PERSON WITH DEMENTIA – EVERYONE'S BUSINESS?

Ideally, ACP should be initiated in primary care as part of the ongoing trusted relationship between GP, nurse and the person with dementia, at a time where there is no crisis element or urgency to act swiftly. In Shiny's case study, both Magda and Oskar missed various opportunities to discuss ACP at the GP practice whilst Magda still had capacity and Oskar was less anxious about his mother's health and wellbeing. Opportunities to commence ACP discussions could have arisen on any number of occasions, such as annual health checks, medication reviews or a yearly invitation for a flu jab. None of these opportunities prompted ACP discussions for Magda, where she could have been signposted to various resources or local services. Oskar, as Magda's main carer, could have spoken to an Admiral Nurse, a Dementia Advisor or any other professional to understand what the benefits of making an LPA and ACP would be. The first admission to hospital should have been seen as a late, but nevertheless key opportunity to initiate an ACP or make it a discharge follow-up action for the GP when Magda returned to the community.

There was clear evidence of rapid deterioration and decline in Magda's overall health with dementia and other co-morbid factors indicating that the best time was 'right there and then'.

Shiny reflected on the readmission and noted that the time had passed where Magda had the ability to engage in discussions about her future care wishes and what would matter to her at the end of her life. Leaving initiating ACP discussions for the acute care setting is a reactive approach since urgent medical treatment and recovery are often prioritized over ACP. Hospital stays in acute wards are usually very short and do not allow enough time for long and frequent ACP discussions to be conducted with trust-building, sensitivity and compassion (NHS 2022). Moreover, it is often unclear who should initiate such discussions, especially since most patients and families are not ready to consider ACP unless prompted over time. Shiny's reflection on Magda's case highlights that the acute ward may not be the optimal environment for ACP discussions. Patients are unwell and may not be able to focus on their future wishes and preferences, and families are often stressed and responding to the immediate crisis situation. These factors reduce the ability to think clearly and sensibly, or make informed decisions for the future when simply worried about what the next day may hold for them.

WHAT ARE THE POTENTIAL BENEFITS TO ACP IN DEMENTIA?

Timely initiation of an ACP discussion has many benefits for the person with dementia, families and health and social care professionals (Harrison Dening et al. 2019; Piers et al. 2018; Tetrault et al. 2022). The person with dementia has an early opportunity to take their time and reflect about what would matter to them as their dementia progresses and they reach the end stages of life. It allows them to make decisions, to speak to their family and supporters, to set up a plan for when they are no longer able to do so. ACP is the time for the person with dementia to voice their wishes and preferences about their future care as part of 'hoping for the best and planning for the worst'. This is a proactive and person-centred approach to care that can lead to a good quality of life by preserving dignity and promoting respect for the individual, their choices, preferences and wishes. Families and people with dementia are happier and more reassured with a firm plan in place where everyone knows what to do in advance and at times where needs change rapidly.

The person with dementia, for example, may prefer wherever possible to stay at home, where they are familiar with their surroundings and surrounded by people who know them well, and not be admitted to hospital. Unnecessary admissions to hospital and treatment escalation are thereby avoided, improving the quality of life for the person with dementia but also reducing the cost impact on health and social care systems. An ACP views dying well as a fully integrated part of living well with dementia.

WHAT COMES UNDER THE UMBRELLA OF ADVANCE CARE PLANNING?

An ACP is a voluntary, personalized and legally binding document that outlines comprehensive and crucial information about a person's future care decisions for when they are no longer able to communicate their wishes or have lost their mental capacity to do so. NHS England in 'My Future Wishes' (NHS 2018), suggests three stages in carrying out ACP discussions:

- **early** (around the time of dementia diagnosis)

- **progressing** (identification of increased care needs)

- **later** (advanced stages of dementia, re-establishing mental capacity and review of anticipatory treatment).

A robust, person-centred ACP should collate information on the following five aspects:

1. Advance Statement: Captures the person's preferred place of care and death. This could be their own home, a care home, a hospital or somewhere else.

2. Advance Decision to Refuse Treatment or Living Will: Reflects a conversation in relation to sudden deterioration or acute illness/abrupt health event (for instance, a fall or myocardial infarction). The person will share their views on whether they would like to be treated at their preferred place of care in terms of three aspects: ventilation (breathing support); treatment (oral or intravenous); and cardio-pulmonary resuscitation.

3. What would matter to the person towards the end stages of their life: Considers the presence of family members, close friends, pets, faith leaders, ethnic and cultural aspects of dying that mean a great deal to the person with dementia. Some people see the end of their life as an opportunity to contribute towards research for a particular disease such as dementia by donating their body to science. However, most people tend to choose either burial or cremation, mostly based on religious or cultural beliefs and traditions.

4. LPA: Indicates the people appointed as decision makers by the person with dementia in the event of mental capacity loss or inability to communicate decisions reliably. There are two strands in LPA: (1) health/welfare; and (2) property/finance. Appointed decision makers could be a family member, a friend, a solicitor or anyone otherwise indicated by the person whilst they still have mental capacity.

5. Funeral arrangements: Sets out any pre-planned or pre-paid arrangements (often as part of a will) so that when the time comes, relatives are spared the stress of deciding what to do on behalf of the deceased. However, not everyone does (or can) plan ahead. Therefore, careful and sensitive consideration is needed when addressing funeral arrangements within ACP discussions as it may confuse or scare patients and families.

CONCLUSION

Talking about death or end of life can be scary and people may fear opening conversations about it. In some cultures, preservation of life matters more than death, whereas in others, death is regarded as a happy day because the dead become liberated from illness, pain, worries and the angst of living. Therefore, it is important that any ACP conversations are held by trained, confident professionals, who are known to the person, and ideally in a place that they are familiar and comfortable with and outside of crisis or intense situations. The person should feel reassured, relaxed and ready to open up more and engage in the ACP discussions.

SOURCES OF SUPPORT

If you have any questions about helping a person with any aspect of dementia, call our free Helpline on 0800 888 6678 or email at helpline@dementiauk.org
If you would prefer a pre-booked appointment by phone or video, call via the Dementia UK website: www.dementiauk.org

RESOURCES

Dementia UK. Planning now for your future – advance care planning. www.dementiauk.org/get-support/legal-and-financial-information/advance-care-planning
Universal Care Plan (London area). https://ucp.onelondon.online/about
Gold Standard Framework – advance care planning (rest of England). www.goldstandardsframework.org.uk/advance-care-planning
Age UK. How to plan ahead for the future with dementia. www.ageuk.org.uk/information-advice/health-wellbeing/conditions-illnesses/dementia/planning-for-the-future
Recommended summary plan for emergency care treatment (ReSPECT). www.resus.org.uk/respect
Admiral Nurse dementia helpline. www.dementiauk.org/get-support/dementia-helpline-alzheimers-helpline

REFERENCES

Detering, K.M., Hancock, A.D., Reade, M.C. et al. (2010) The impact of advance care planning on end-of-life care in elderly patients: Randomised controlled trial. *BMJ*. 340: c1345. https://doi.org/10.1136/bmj.c1345
DH (2008) *End of life care strategy.* https://assets.publishing.service.gov.uk/government/uploads/system/uploads/attachment_data/file/136431/End_of_life_strategy.pdf

Harrison Dening, K., Sampson, E.L. & De Vries, K. (2019) Advance care planning in dementia: Recommendations for healthcare professionals. *Palliative Care.* 12: https://doi.org/10.1177/1178224219826579

NHS (2020) *NHS health check.* www.nhs.uk/conditions/nhs-health-check

NHS (2022) *Universal principles for advance care planning.* www.england.nhs.uk/wp-content/uploads/2022/03/universal-principles-for-advance-care-planning.pdf

NHS England (2018) *My future wishes: Advance care planning (ACP) for people with dementia in all care settings.* www.england.nhs.uk/publication/my-future-wishes-advance-care-planning-acp-for-people-with-dementia-in-all-care-settings

NICE (2018) Dementia: Assessment, management and support for people living with dementia and their carers. NICE guideline [NG97]. www.nice.org.uk/guidance/ng97

Office for National Statistics (ONS) (2020) *Dementia and Alzheimer's disease deaths including comorbidities, England and Wales: 2019 registrations.* www.ons.gov.uk/peoplepopulationandcommunity/birthsdeathsandmarriages/deaths/bulletins/dementiaandalzheimersdiseasedeathsincludingcomorbiditieseng landandwales/2019registrations

Piers, R., Albers, G., Gilissen, J. *et al.* (2018) Advance care planning in dementia: Recommendations for healthcare professionals. *BMC Palliative Care.* 17: 88. https://doi.org/10.1186/s12904-018-0332-2

Tetrault, A., Nyback, M.H., Vaartio-Rajalin, H. et al. (2022) Advance care planning in dementia care: Wants, beliefs, and insight. *Nursing Ethics.* 29(3): 696–708.

CHAPTER 17

Dying with or from dementia

END-OF-LIFE CARE CAN BE COMPLEX

INTRODUCTION

Dementia has not traditionally been conceptualized as a terminal or life-limiting condition. Yet dementia can significantly reduce a person's survival time from the onset of symptoms and has been shown to be similar to that of some cancers. Identifying when a person with dementia is reaching the end of their life can be challenging. Numerous studies have attempted to identify prognostic indicators or indices that may guide clinicians in adopting a more palliative approach to care, but these tools have often been found to be more reliable at identifying people with dementia at low risk of dying rather than those at higher risk of death.

This case study tells us of Alan, who had both cancer and dementia and was admitted to hospice care for management of his symptoms. Whilst some people with a diagnosis of dementia may live into the very advanced stages of dementia and die from their dementia, many more die from another co-morbid life-limiting illness in addition to their dementia. The dementia specialist nurse (Admiral Nurse) then discusses how a person can die with or from dementia and how we can both recognize the signs when a person with dementia is reaching the end of their life and how best to manage the symptoms.

**Elizabeth Jenkins, Palliative Care
Nurse, The Myton Hospices**

The human mind and body are complex. End-of-life care can be complex. During my career in palliative care, I have come to appreciate this in ever-increasing degrees. Caring for people at the end of their lives has been the main focus of my professional career. We, as specialist palliative care practitioners, have become adept at prognosticating the final months, weeks, days and hours of life for those in our care. Admittedly with fluctuating degrees of accuracy but nevertheless with reasonable confidence and aptitude.

Be that as it may, individuals with dementia as a co-morbidity, or indeed as a singular morbidity, present new challenges to this clinical judgement. As a nurse on an inpatient unit within a local 20-bed hospice I can reflect upon the care we provided to one gentleman in particular.

Alan, age 89 years, was admitted onto the hospice inpatient unit with cancer of his prostate and a co-morbidity of Alzheimer's disease. Coupled with his diagnoses, he was predictably frail, weak, was experiencing poor appetite and sleep, breathlessness and occasional abdominal pain. His cancer had been relatively well controlled over recent years and there were no other presenting ailments that were likely to lead him into his last days.

Alan became increasingly unkempt on the ward as he declined frequent offers of assistance to provide personal hygiene; his already waning appetite now saw him eating only morsels of jelly and the occasional spoonful of soup. His mind, however, seemed activated by storytelling and assertions of going on holiday and the need to pack a suitcase, or visiting the post office. He became agitated in the late afternoon, often proceeding into nights that were fraught with his requests to 'remove men from his room' that only he could see and a determination to vacate his bed despite the incapacity of his legs. The questions presenting to the clinical team were ones surrounding separating the predictable patterns of end of life in cancer and those of end of life in dementia.

What was causing his deterioration? What could be done to ease his mental distress? What were the determining factors in symptom control and anticipatory prescribing? Was this gentleman dying? Was he dying of dementia? Was he dying of cancer? What could we do to ease his suffering? The latter question is at the heart of all palliative care practices: What is my role in lessening the suffering of others?

Over the course of a few weeks, however, staff became familiar with his behaviour and felt better equipped to support and care for Alan. The clinical team began to see that the periods of hallucinations were no longer predictable in the latter parts of the day, rather presenting more consistently across the span of the shifts. He continued to decline personal care but was less resistant to prompts to remain in his bed or chair, seemingly becoming moribund and emotionally vacant. Such observations aided our identification that he was entering his final days of life. Proficient communications skills were required to inform and prepare his family members for what was to come, which proved especially difficult as the family had expected death on several occasions before, only for Alan to stabilize and live on. Professionals need to demonstrate confidence to predict and prognosticate end of life, all the while allowing room for an element of uncertainty. The challenges patients with dementia present can compound this judgement. There are blurred lines between refractory delirium and hallucinations manifesting from dementia, similarly the retraction from social interaction, withdrawal from the desire to eat and drink, prominence of compromised tissue viability, immobility and the increase in sleeping and despondency cross between the two presentations of both cancer and dementia. It seemed that whilst Alan's diagnosis of cancer may well have aided his entryway into palliative care and subsequently the hospice setting, in actual fact it was his dementia that triggered most of his uncontrolled symptoms. The question then evolves, do we treat him as though he is dying of cancer or dementia? Is this distinction important or even necessary?

The pathway of dying from malignancy can feel familiar and even safer to anticipate for palliative care clinicians; dementia is much less predictable and quantifiable. End of life for those with a dementia diagnosis can often be confused with temporary declines in health which may have been frequent occurrences for family and loved ones to observe prior to this moment. Sometimes it takes professional skill and confidence to identify when this is not the case and in fact the individual is actively dying.

Sharron Tolman, Academy Lead Admiral Nurse

Elizabeth raises some very important issues in considering end of life in people with dementia. One-third of people aged over 65 will die with or from dementia (Brayne et al. 2006), now the commonest cause of death in the UK. By 2040 it is estimated that 220,000 people per year will die with dementia in England and Wales, with many experiencing distressing symptoms like pain and agitation requiring palliative care. Although dementia mainly affects people over the age of 60, it is not a normal part of ageing (WHO and Alzheimer's Disease International 2012).

DIAGNOSTIC OVERSHADOWING OF DEMENTIA

Dementia has become the most feared and stigmatized condition over cancer, which can often lead to negative outcomes for people with dementia and their families due to the effect of overshadowing that their dementia diagnosis can have over their other conditions. This, and limited understanding of dementia as a neurodegenerative life-limiting condition, impacts on the experiences of families affected by dementia towards end of life. Changes in symptoms may simply be attributed to the progression of dementia, rather than recognizing the possibility of the person moving towards end of life. This might have been the case with Alan in the early days of his admission to the hospice, but staff developed an understanding of Alan and patterns in his presentation and adjusted their care and support in a person-centred way. However, end of life in dementia remains poorly defined, so there is a need to move beyond simply a focus on cognitive and functional decline to a more needs-based approach, which is not based on the stage of dementia (Browne et al. 2021).

DYING WITH OR FROM DEMENTIA?

People may die of other illnesses in the earlier stages of dementia before they reach later or end stages, and this would seem to be the case with Alan in respect of his co-morbid diagnosis of cancer. Nevertheless, one-third of people with dementia will live into its advanced stages (Sleeman et al. 2019), though commonly living with multi-morbidities. With delays in diagnosis, the time from diagnosis to death may also be more uncertain or misleading if symptoms began many years prior to a formal diagnosis. Therefore, as Elizabeth describes, recognizing when someone with dementia may be in the last phase of their life can be complex.

The trajectory of dementia is often slow with periods of worsening health then episodes of recovery, and Elizabeth alludes to this. Managing uncertainty is typical with this unpredictable trajectory. People with dementia often experience a high symptom burden, not dissimilar to those experienced by people in the advanced stages of cancer, such as pain, breathing difficulties, swallowing difficulties and constipation. However, these symptoms are less likely to be recognized and receive appropriate care and treatment and equitable access to palliative care; in Alan's case, his admission to the hospice was based on his cancer diagnosis not his dementia diagnosis.

Palliative care traditionally may be required at times of deteriorating health, change or uncertainty, but with dementia a palliative approach is recommended from diagnosis to offer people living with dementia flexible needs based care that considers how unpredictable dementia can be (NICE 2018). However, ongoing monitoring and review of a person following a diagnosis of dementia is limited in health and social care; this results in less opportunity to pick up on changes or signs of when a person is moving towards their end of life. Relieving suffering, which may be physical, psychological, social or spiritual, with the need for palliative care to improve quality of life, maximize function and comfort at **all** stages of dementia, is essential. As Elizabeth describes, Alan was experiencing a range of symptoms, such as delirium, reduced mobility and appetite, reduced ability to communicate, increasing withdrawal, sleepiness and skin changes which are all common symptoms towards end of life generally and similarly so in dementia. These symptoms can often be misunderstood and drive crisis admissions into acute hospital care, with a sharp rise in Emergency Department attendances in the last 12 months of life for people with dementia (Yorganci et al. 2022), rather than care that is in line with their palliative care needs.

DYING WITH DEMENTIA

Public Health England have developed a framework and set of recommendations to guide clinical practice to ensure that all people who are dying receive high-quality, compassionate and joined-up care (PHE 2019). These include person-centred care, communication and shared decision making, optimal treatment of symptoms and providing comfort, setting care goals, advance planning, continuity of care, psychosocial and spiritual support, family care and involvement, nutrition and hydration, prognostication and timely recognition of dying.

There are measures such as the Integrated Palliative Outcome Scale for people with dementia (IPOS-Dem), a holistic measure designed specifically for dementia to help recognize when a need for palliative care emerges in routine care or in any setting. The IPOS-Dem measure can support assessing and managing symptoms which may be causing distress, with a focus on monitoring the symptoms and concerns important to the person with dementia and their family over time. Picking up on symptoms even in earlier stages of dementia, such as pain, loss of appetite and mobility changes, loss of interest in activities, anxiety and family carer distress, is important for many reasons. Early identification and management can contribute to a person's wellbeing, identify when concerns need to be escalated, help to decide priorities in care, support record keeping and open up communication and collaboration between the multi-disciplinary team and family living with dementia. In addition, the use of IPOS-Dem has been shown to support the education of health and social care professionals, and enhance decision making and person-centred care, seeing the person behind the dementia.

Using the IPOS-Dem measure with Alan may have supported earlier identification and association of his issues with dementia, enabling professionals to be more aware of the changes in his presentation and the possibility of the transition towards end of life. Similarly, registering a person with dementia on a Palliative Care Register within primary care (see an example of an explanatory leaflet in the Resources section) can also be used to support ongoing monitoring so the changes are picked up, increasing the likelihood of identifying the transition towards end of life and dying.

RECOGNIZING DELIRIUM TOWARDS THE END OF LIFE IN A PERSON WITH DEMENTIA

Sometimes health and social care professionals, and indeed family carers, may find it difficult to understand how to care for and treat a person with dementia. As in Alan's case, the staff caring for him were seeking to understand if his needs were different. Did they require a different approach? Alan probably was experiencing a delirium superimposed on his dementia, which is common towards end of life. When Elizabeth and the team questioned how to ease Alan's distress, considering delirium seemed a significant factor, with Alan experiencing symptoms such as hallucinations and distressing ideas of intruders in his hospice room. As hallucinations, perceptual problems and paranoid ideas can occur at different stages of the condition, delirium is often missed towards the end of life.

There is also the challenge with terminology and language, with a variety of words used to describe delirium, such as confusion, agitation, sundowning and, in the dying phase, terminal agitation and terminal restlessness. This variation can compound the challenge of diagnosing and managing delirium well and addressing any other underlying symptoms which may be contributing to the delirium such as pain, constipation, medication and the environment. Working with Alan and his family to establish an understanding of his previous baseline and what is normal or usual for him would be key. If delirium is explained to families, apart from offering some reassurance that professionals know what is happening, it may also improve their wellbeing and confidence to understand what is happening and help them to contribute to non-pharmacological strategies to reduce Alan's distress. This may include responding to changes in perceptions and hallucinations calmly, avoiding disagreeing with what Alan is experiencing (as this is very real for him) by acknowledging how upsetting this must be for him, and offering reassurance and any distractions to ease his distress. The family can also support Alan with orientation and ensure he is wearing glasses and hearing aids as required.

CAPACITY AND DECISION MAKING

There is also the issue of capacity. Compared to other conditions, a neurodegenerative disorder such as dementia is more likely to impact on a person's capacity to make choices and decisions. When caring for a person with dementia, families often describe feeling ill-equipped and poorly prepared, with proxy decision making a significant source of distress for them. Assessing Alan's capacity, under the principles of the Mental Capacity Act 2005, to make decisions about his care involves giving him every opportunity to communicate. Even in the advanced stages of dementia there are still ways of enabling communication, for example with communication cards or other means of non-verbal communication, to enable choice and expression of needs, which may rely less on verbal skills. Can Alan understand information given to him? Can he retain it long enough to be able to make the decision? Can he weigh up the information available to make the decision and can he communicate his decision? Are there any other ways we can help Alan to express his needs and wishes?

If Alan was assessed as not having mental capacity, decisions may need to be made in his best interests. Family carers and supporters and all staff involved in his care are pivotal in any best interest decision and making the process and the outcomes person-centred. This involves understanding Alan's history, lifestyle, interests, culture and preferences and what needs to be known for his individualized comfort care planning. Questions that might also be considered are:

- What gives Alan emotional and physical comfort?

- What makes Alan feel safe and comfortable, relaxed, happy and pain free?

The argument for early advance planning before capacity is lost gives the person with dementia the opportunity to express preferences, wishes and choices which may be helpful in enabling the best interest decision-making process. For example, how could Alan communicate his needs early to reduce distress later? How can his physical, psychological, spiritual and social 'pain' be met with a progressive illness and changing needs? Opportunities to support Alan and his family to explore this during the trajectory of dementia and consider contingency planning may support shared decision making at end of life and potentially minimize guilt and distress for the family making decisions on his behalf.

MANY FELT LOSSES

Towards end of life, families have often been caring for the person with dementia for many years, living with the uncertainty and unpredictability. It is likely they have experienced several distressing transitions and made difficult decisions, often in times of crisis. Grief and loss are hugely significant factors throughout the trajectory of dementia which need to be considered. For the person with dementia, this may include loss of independence, roles and identity, social connection, memory, relationships, control, physical abilities, skills, communication, home, friends and family. For the family, losses may include the relationship they had with the person before the diagnosis of dementia, changing roles, intimacy, a shared future, connection, shared interests, lifestyle and social life. Family carers also can experience anticipatory grief that is felt before the person with dementia dies. This form of grief and loss may go unrecognized and can lead to an increase in the risk of depression. Ambiguous loss may also be a factor, with carers having a sense of the person with dementia being absent and present at the same time, living with a lack of solution, difficulty in knowing how to grieve, with loss affecting coping behaviours.

So, thinking about Alan and his family, what losses have they experienced or are experiencing? How is this impacting on them now? Can we support this family during the trajectory of dementia to understand the impact of grief and loss and adapt communication styles to enable the person affected by dementia to express themselves? This may be about giving time to process, checking understanding, validating emotion and chunking information and/or using creative outlets through reminiscence, music or art.

PLACE OF DEATH

Only about 6% of people with dementia die in their own home, with most dying in a care home (PHE 2019). There are likely multiple reasons for this but including end-of-life conversations in more routine dementia care, when the person with dementia is still living at home, can open up opportunities to discuss death and dying. Many people with dementia, when given a diagnosis of dementia, are often not given any information on their prognosis and what to expect as the condition progresses. As with any life-limiting condition people need to understand what they need to consider when thinking about their future preferences and wishes for care. Similarly, providing family carers and supporters with explanations to support their understanding of changes they may encounter is important. This can include why is the person eating and drinking less, why are they experiencing swallowing problems, repeated infections, responding less to treatment? Communicating clearly and expanding explanations beyond it simply being about the 'dementia progression' to the person possibly being in the last months/year of their life will influence decisions about care and, in some instances, enable more choice in place of death.

CONCLUSION

This chapter has considered how health and social care staff can provide a palliative approach to dementia from early diagnosis, which may contribute to more timely recognition of end-of-life care needs and an improved end-of-life experience for the person with dementia and their family carers. Recognizing end of life can be difficult and may lead to fewer people with dementia accessing specialist palliative care services and hospices, therefore proactive assessment, management and monitoring of physical, psychological, social and spiritual needs is essential within routine care to recognize end of life.

SOURCES OF SUPPORT

If you have any questions about helping a person with any aspect of dementia, call our free Helpline on 0800 888 6678 or email at helpline@dementiauk.org
If you would prefer a pre-booked appointment by phone or video, call via the Dementia UK website: www.dementiauk.org

RESOURCES

UCL. **Supporting you to make decisions while caring for someone living with dementia during Coronavirus (COVID-19) and beyond.** www.ucl.ac.uk/psychiatry/research/marie-curie-palliative-care-research-department/research/decision-aid

Rules of thumb: End-of-life care for people with dementia. www.ucl.ac.uk/epidemiology-health-care/sites/epidemiology-health-care/files/demenita_rot.pdf

Eating and drinking: Information for family and friends as dementia progresses towards the end of life. https://hukstage-new-bucket.s3.eu-west-2.amazonaws.com/s3fs-public/2022-11/eating-and-drinking-final.pdf

IPOS-Dem. https://pos-pal.org/maix/ipos-dem.php

Six Steps. Six steps to success in end of life care. https://eolp.co.uk/SIXSTEPS

Dementia toolkit: Living your life with hope. Dealing with grief and loss. https://livingwithdementiatoolkit.org.uk/stay-positive/dealing-with-grief-and-loss

NHS England. Example of an explanatory leaflet. www.england.nhs.uk/northwest/wp-content/uploads/sites/48/2021/11/EPaCCS-Patient-Information-trifold-V1.4-reviewed-June2020.pdf

REFERENCES

Brayne, C., Gao, L. & Dewey, M. (2006) Medical Research Council cognitive function and ageing study investigators: Dementia before death in ageing societies – the promise of prevention and the reality. *PLoS Medicine*. 3(10): e397. https://doi:10.1371/journal.pmed.0030397

Browne, B., Kupeli, N., Moore, K. et al. (2021) Defining end of life in dementia: A systematic review. *Palliative Medicine*. 35(10). https://doi.org/10.1177/026921632110254

Mental Capacity Act (2005) www.legislation.gov.uk/ukpga/2005/9/contents

National Institute for Health and Care Excellence (NICE) (2018) *Dementia: Assessment, management and support for people living with dementia and their carers (Guideline NG97)*. www.nice.org.uk/guidance/ng97

PHE (2019) *PHE strategy 2020 to 2025*. www.gov.uk/government/publications/phe-strategy-2020-to-2025

Sleeman, K.E., de Brito, M., Etkind, S. et al. (2019) The escalating global burden of serious health-related suffering: Projections to 2060 by world regions, age groups, and health conditions. *The Lancet: Global Health*. 7(7): e883–e892. https://doi:10.1016/S2214-109X(19)30172-X

World Health Organization and Alzheimer's Disease International (2012) *Dementia: A public health priority*. https://iris.who.int/bitstream/handle/10665/75263/9789241564458_eng.pdf?sequence=1

Yorganci, E., Stewart, R., Sampson, E.L. et al. (2022) Patterns of unplanned hospital admissions among people with dementia: From diagnosis to the end of life. *Age and Ageing*. 51(5): afac098. https://doi.org/10.1093/ageing/afac098

CHAPTER 18

Gaps in care and support provision

INTRODUCTION

There are significant gaps in the provision of health and social care support for people with dementia and their families. Increasingly, charitable and not-for-profit organizations are left to fill these gaps.

Getting a diagnosis can be difficult due to a lack of awareness of the early signs and symptoms of dementia (see also Chapter 2), not just by the person who is symptomatic, but also their family, friends, colleagues and health and social care staff. There is also still a fear about what a diagnosis could mean and what changes may be necessary, and this can lead to a reluctance to come forward for an assessment. The waiting list for a diagnostic assessment of dementia also extends the time before an accurate diagnosis can be given.

Once the diagnosis is received, however, families often report that there is little in the way of post-diagnostic support for the person diagnosed or the rest of the family, with an over-reliance on giving out leaflets which families report can be overwhelming and not focusing on what they need to do now.

There are also financial costs associated with a diagnosis of dementia, for example loss of employment, care, and support costs, and in some cases payment for a private assessment if the waiting list is too long. There are frequently families who do not receive the necessary financial support and advice to help them to cope with these costs (Kilty et al. 2023).

Alison Stewart writes about her personal experience of supporting her mother with dementia and the gaps in service and support she experienced. She also writes about the Memory Hubs she supports in

Northamptonshire, the work she does for the Academy for Dementia Research and Education, and includes the experiences of the gaps in provision for the families who attend and how this impacts them. Following this a dementia specialist nurse (Admiral Nurse) responds with advice on supporting families with dementia to navigate these gaps.

Alison Stewart, Memory Hub Manager, West Northamptonshire

In 2016, I secured a promoted teaching post in further education. I had worked hard as a mature student and widowed parent to gain higher qualifications and reach this point, but I was also increasingly aware of my mum's declining health. She had become heavily reliant on my support and her change of character, though subtle at first, meant that she gradually became much more demanding of me. We reached a crisis point when I was in the first term of a new teaching post and, no longer able to juggle my working hours with my mum's care, I regrettably handed in my notice. In hindsight, perhaps if I was more informed about dementia or had someone been available to talk to about its impact on my work, I might have discussed options rather than lose a career and income.

It was my lived experience of dementia that led me to work for a University of Northampton research project called UnityDem. The project offered early intervention support for people recently diagnosed with dementia and my role was to offer social interaction activities with a focus on cognitive stimulation and light physical activity.

I now facilitate early intervention activity groups for people recently diagnosed with dementia and their selected family member. It's a privileged position but I am also acutely aware of service gaps in the system.

Worrying about finances and needing appropriate advice is common in our groups, especially with younger families who are not yet at retirement age. For example, some families are bearing the costs of caring for the person with dementia by giving up their own careers. A wife told me: 'We put so much work into our family "forever home" but we had to sell it to manage.' A widowed husband diagnosed with dementia told me: 'They can take all you have worked for over the years, everything you own if you get worse and have to go into care.'

The common experience I hear throughout the groups is that after diagnosis, some people feel they are 'Left to our own devices' or 'Dumped.' Most describe the pile of leaflets they receive that can often be overwhelming. There is some useful literature but with so much information, 'It's hard to know where to begin.'

Sometimes individuals are referred to websites and electronic forms but often these are unfamiliar or inaccessible without the ownership and regular use of modern technology. Even the terminology used by local services can be confusing. Some organizations or support groups have similar names and it's hard to differentiate what specific support they provide. If someone has savings beyond the threshold of £23,250, they are classed as a 'self-funder' and therefore handed a directory of care services to contact independently.

'Care assessment' and 'care package' are terms often used by different service providers but not necessarily understood by service users; What do these mean and what do they provide in practical terms? The various financial allowances that are available are a mystery to most and the process for applying, understanding whether they are means tested or require the completion of lengthy forms, is often too onerous. One of our determined members took her form and supporting documents to be helped in person by a service provider but was told she did not qualify for the allowance, only to find later that she was given the wrong advice and was in fact eligible for financial support. She received the correct advice from a peer. People with dementia and their families need proficient guidance and consistency of advice from service providers.

Even the basic understanding of what dementia means and an individual's specific diagnosis can cause stress and confusion. For example, some people ask what the difference is between dementia and Alzheimer's (dementia is an umbrella term whilst Alzheimer's is a specific diagnosis) and understandably only know the sensationalized stories told in the media or dramatized on television: 'I don't know what type of dementia they have', said one wife. 'I just know it's dementia!'

We have seen confidence grow when members develop tools through informal training and looking at their experience through a different perspective. Perhaps the most beneficial experience is having time bonding with group members and gaining knowledge through peer support. During one of my 'Brain Gym' groups, a small group of wives who support husbands diagnosed with dementia meet every week in a café next door. They have become a support network for each other, sharing practical, financial and emotional advice. After all, they are the experts! This exceptional peer group needed the facility of space and reassurance that their loved ones with dementia were being supported next door. Caregivers who support loved ones with dementia are short on time and space to be independent. It is almost impossible to ensure self-care. Members describe our groups as the 'Highlight of our week' or a 'lifeline'. That's not to say we don't sometimes share tears and frustrations.

Working with younger people diagnosed with dementia (before 65 years) has presented additional concerns and gaps in the system. There are more financial implications due to the loss of work and income. Sometimes there are children still at home who become young carers: 'Support groups are during the day when my children are at school, and I am at work.' We need more age-appropriate groups that address the needs and interests of younger families. One concerned mother told me that she lies awake at night worrying about her son who lives alone and was diagnosed with frontotemporal dementia in his 50s. There was a query on his Personal Independence Payment and because he was unable to answer questions on the phone, he lost the payment and is still trying to reapply a year later. Services need to be much more aware of dementia and have informed advocates available.

Supporting family members, even with Lasting Power of Attorney, can be exhausting and still problematic. Hospital appointments and visiting rights are a worrying issue for several of our members. Even after COVID restrictions relaxed, people with dementia staying in hospital were often not permitted visitors despite having Lasting Power of Attorney for Health and Wellbeing. My mum spent days on a hospital trolley in A&E without appropriate care. I received a phone call in the middle of the night to say: 'Can you tell us what's wrong? She seems a bit confused.' She had advanced dementia and was at end of life. It took days of impassioned phone calls to gain palliative care and access for the family. We shouldn't need to fight for appropriate care.

Laura Birch, Admiral Nurse Dementia Resource Community

In this case study, Alison Stewart highlights her experience in relation to caring for her mother living with dementia and the experience of the attendees at the Memory Hub. Alison identifies common themes such as getting a diagnosis, trying to balance work and caring responsibilities, barriers after diagnosis and difficulties accessing financial support.

GAPS IN GETTING A DIAGNOSIS

Alison identifies her mother's personality changes and reliance on her for care needs as early indicators of her mother's dementia. Dementia can present with varied symptoms, each diagnosis unique to the individual, causing difficulties in obtaining a timely diagnosis. This is more apparent with young onset dementia because often the early signs and symptoms can mimic other conditions including depression or burnout (Perry et al. 2023). In addition, there may be a reluctance to seek an assessment and diagnosis due to denial of the early symptoms, and fear of getting diagnosed with dementia (Parker et al. 2020).

Timely diagnosis of dementia is vital to initiating appropriate support, for the individual living with dementia and their caregivers. Without timely support, from the beginning of diagnosis, individuals can often feel lost and left to navigate health and social care services as indicated by the group that Alison facilitates.

GAPS IN SUPPORT FOR WORKING CARERS

There are identifiable gaps in support, especially for working carers, who have difficulties in managing their working life, and providing care support to their family member. This was identified by Alison and led to her leaving the employment she trained for. Support at this stage could have prevented this but often workplace knowledge on dementia and its perceived challenges are low, leading to a lack of understanding and support and the potential need for flexible working arrangements (Carers UK 2014). Carers UK (2014) identified that both employers and employees identified the need for clearer, more accessible information on dementia, the need for a wider understanding of the added responsibilities and the need for flexibility for those employees who are caring for a family member. The report also emphasized that the key role of employers is to support their colleagues within this situation, providing an inclusive culture.

After COVID-19, many organizations moved to more flexible ways of working, including working from home, flexitime and job sharing. This may enable carers to manage their workload and caring duties more effectively. However, working from home may give rise to additional problems for the family carer who used to like going to a workplace to have time away from caring responsibilities.

GAPS IN PROVIDING INFORMATION ABOUT FINANCES AND BENEFITS

Following a diagnosis of dementia, individuals are often encouraged to explore financial support and benefits. Advice and guidance on claiming benefits and financial support can often be inconsistent, due to some being means tested and some requiring certain criteria be met, which can cause confusion for caregivers. The groups that Alison facilitates were vocal about the problems and perceived lack of fairness about the provision of financial support and benefits when a family member has dementia. These financial issues are particularly acute for younger people living with dementia (Bayly et al. 2021) with families identifying that leaving employment early impacts not just on the person diagnosed but their whole family.

There are two main benefits that can be claimed by people diagnosed with dementia:

1. Personal Independent Payment (PIP) is a benefit which can be applied for by individuals living with young onset dementia, i.e., dementia under the age of 65 years. There are two parts to PIP, a daily living part which assesses if the person living with dementia needs help with everyday tasks, and a mobility part which assesses if the individual needs help moving around.

2. Attendance Allowance (AA) is a benefit that can be claimed by people diagnosed with dementia over 65 years of age. AA helps with extra costs if the person has a disability severe enough that they need someone to help look after them. AA is paid

at two different rates depending on the level of care that is needed.

Once the individual completes their application, they may be required to include details of which professionals support the individual living with dementia, e.g., a GP or health and social care professional. The Department of Work and Pensions will assess the application to establish if the individual meets the criteria, such as their level of difficulty at completing daily living- or mobility-based tasks. In addition to the above benefits the person living with dementia may be entitled to a council tax reduction depending on who lives in the home and other benefits claimed.

Carers of those living with dementia may be entitled to the Carer's Allowance; this may entitle the carer to receive a weekly sum of money if they care for the person with dementia for at least 35 hours a week, and the person with dementia gets certain benefits. This benefit is means tested and varies depending on the person's earnings.

Local support services, including third sector organizations, can provide guidance and assistance applying for these benefits and financial support options, however availability can vary depending on locality due to gaps in service provision.

GAPS IN POST-DIAGNOSTIC SUPPORT, INCLUDING INFORMATION NEEDS AND NAVIGATING THE HEALTH AND SOCIAL CARE SYSTEM

After receiving a diagnosis of dementia, it can be difficult to navigate the health and social care system, especially if the person is under the age of 65 years. This is due to a lack of age-appropriate activities and support being available, as many groups are tailored to people over the age of 65 years. Alison indicates that for the groups she facilitates there is a feeling that after diagnosis and after being given leaflets, there is very little post-diagnostic support available, regardless of age.

Family carers are entitled to a 'Carers Assessment' which identifies the carer's needs, and the impact caring responsibilities have on their life. From this assessment support needs are identified which, if addressed, will enable the carer to continue their role. This could include accessing respite care, help from home carers, or equipment or support for the carer's mental wellbeing. The person with dementia is also entitled to an 'Adult Needs Assessment' which identifies their needs, including activities of daily living, and identifies support that would be appropriate to improve their physical, intellectual, emotional and social wellbeing. Often health and social care professionals do not alert the family living with dementia to the availability of these assessments or how to access them.

Admiral Nurses can help support families who are experiencing difficulty in accessing appropriate post-diagnostic support. This includes information on finances, employment and strategies to reduce distress caused by difficult symptoms. Admiral Nurses provide specialist dementia advice and support to families living with the impact of dementia and to health and social care professionals, who may need advice and support with issues that may arise within their practice regarding dementia.

THE ROLE OF THIRD SECTOR ORGANIZATIONS AND PEER SUPPORT IN BRIDGING THESE GAPS AND WHERE TO FIND INFORMATION ABOUT WHAT IS AVAILABLE

In their study, Bamford et al. (2021) identified that there are five key themes of post-diagnostic support: timely identification and management of needs; understanding and managing dementia; emotional and psychological wellbeing; practical support; and integrating support. Families report that following diagnosis, frequently post-diagnostic support is limited or non-existent, as also evidenced in Alison's case study. Third sector organizations, including peer support programmes, attempt to bridge the gaps in service provision for those living with dementia and their families. These can often include day care settings, providing respite to carers, and meaningful interventions and social engagement for those living with dementia. This aims to bring people together, providing social support and guidance within a relaxed environment.

The support available will vary depending on the local area. Many localities have support in the form of 'Dementia Cafés' or 'Memory Hubs', where the person living with dementia and their carer or family can attend with them to gain social support, advice and guidance from local professionals who may also attend these groups. In the locality in which I work, there are a variety of local groups, from singing groups, to fitness groups, and groups that go on different days out, varying each month. These are organized by non-profit and third sector organizations aiming to make a difference.

It can sometimes be difficult to establish what support there is in the local area; sometimes social prescribers have a list of local social groups. Age UK and the Alzheimer's Society have websites which give details of local services on entering a postcode. These sites do not indicate where specialist dementia nurse (Admiral Nurse) services are, however these can be found via the Admiral Nurse Dementia Helpline.

CONCLUSION

It is important to recognize that needs will vary, depending on individual preferences. Therefore, gaining a history of the individual living with dementia and their carer and establishing what support they may require is important. Gaps in services will remain, and identifying these gaps will enable us to understand and provide support that is not currently in place.

SOURCES OF SUPPORT

If you have any questions about helping a person with any aspect of dementia, call our free Helpline on 0800 888 6678 or email at helpline@dementiauk.org
If you would prefer a pre-booked appointment by phone or video, call via the Dementia UK website: www.dementiauk.org

REFERENCES

Bamford, C., Wheatley, A., Brunskill, G. et al. (2021) Key components of post-diagnostic support for people with dementia and their carers: A qualitative study. *PloS One.* 16(12): e0260506. https://doi:10.1371/journal.pone.0260506
Bayly, M., O'Connell, M.E., Kortzman, A. et al. (2021) Family carers' narratives of the financial consequences of young onset dementia. *Dementia.* 20(8): 2708–2724.
Carers UK (2014) *Supporting employees who are caring for someone with dementia.* www.dementiaaction.org.uk/assets/0000/9168/Supporting_employees_who_are_caring_for_someone_with_dementia.pdf

Kilty, C., Cahill, S., Foley, T. et al. (2023) Young onset dementia: Implications for employment and finances. *Dementia.* 22(1): 68–84.

Parker, M., Barlow, S., Hoe, J. et al. (2020) Persistent barriers and facilitators to seeking help for a dementia diagnosis: A systematic review of 30 years of the perspectives of carers and people with dementia. *International Psychogeriatrics.* 32(5): 611–634.

Perry, M., Michgelsen, J., Timmers, R. et al. (2023) Perceived barriers and solutions by generalist physicians to work towards timely young-onset dementia diagnosis. *Aging & Mental Health.* https://doi:10.1080/13607863.2023.2248026

Index

221

King's Fund 125
Kitwood, T. 67, 89, 112, 119

language issues
as symptom of dementia 35
Levy, Joseph 17
Liddle, J. 159
life story work 80–1
Lillo-Crespo, M. 125
'lived in' domiciliary care
case studies on 132–3
challenges of 133–5
communication in 138
and discomfort 137–8
eating and drinking 138–9
and pain 137–8
personal care in 136–7
liver function
as mimicking symptom 36
Lord, S.R. 165
losing things
as symptom of dementia 35
lost, getting
case studies on 86–8
impacts of 85–6
and Mental Capacity Act 91–2
and risk management 88–9
and risk prevention 92–4
and risk taking 89–90
safeguarding 90–1
as symptom of dementia 35

MacKay, Anthony
on falls 164–5
Manning, S.N. 107
Mantle, R. 86, 89
McDermott, O. 101
memory loss
and community nursing 146–7
as symptom of dementia 34, 35
Mental Capacity Act (2005)
44–5, 56, 91–2, 93–4, 113,
126, 138, 148, 206
Mills, R. 46
mimicking symptoms of
dementia 35–7

Mitchell, Wendy 55
mood changes
as symptom of dementia 35
Montgomery, P. 85
Morandi, A. 120
Morris, L. 75
multi-disciplinary working 47–9
'My Future Wishes' (NHS) 194

National Health Service
(NHS) 191, 193, 194
National Institute for Health &
Care Excellence (NICE) 38,
92, 122, 127, 165, 166, 191, 203
National Institute for Health and
Care Research (NIHR) 60
National Police Improve-
ment Agency 85
NHS RightCare 119
Nolan, M. 134
non-verbal communication 70–2

Office for Health Improvement
and Disparities (OHID) 166
Office for National Sta-
tistics (ONS) 191
Oliver, Keith 11
O'Reilly, Melissa
on Emergency Department
(ED) treatment 108–9
O'Shea, E. 82

pain 137–8
Pain Assessment in Advanced
Dementia (PAINAD) 137
Parker, M. 215
Parveen, S. 19
patient assessments in Emergency
Departments 110–11
Pepper, A. 67, 72, 110
Perry, M. 215
Perry-Young, L. 39
person-centred commu-
nication 67–9
personality changes
as symptom of dementia 35

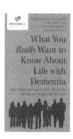

What You Really Want to Know About Life with Dementia: Real stories and expert advice for family, friends and people with dementia

Karen Harrison Dening, Hilda Hayo and Christine Reddall. Foreword by Keith Oliver

A family-led vision of what carers of people with dementia need and want to know. Supporting families and carers in their day-to-day life with dementia, this unique resource combines real stories from families with expert responses and advice for specific issues and concerns.

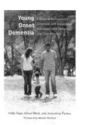

Young Onset Dementia: A Guide to Recognition, Diagnosis, and Supporting Individuals with Dementia and Their Families

Hilda Hayo, Alison Ward, and Jacqueline Parkes. Foreword by Wendy Mitchell

Highlighting the importance of timely recognition and diagnosis of young onset dementia, this book considers the interventions, services and support available to individuals and their families, with practical steps for improving practice. Lived experiences of people with young onset dementia are included alongside learning points.

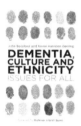

Dementia, Culture and Ethnicity: Issues for All

Edited by Julia Botsford and Karen Harrison Dening. Foreword by Alistair Burns

This book explores the relationship between dementia, culture and ethnicity, looking at the latest evidence and research to determine the impact of diversity on dementia care services. By examining the key issues and providing suggestions for change, this book shows how dementia professionals can provide culturally appropriate care for all.

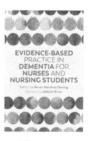

Evidence-Based Practice in Dementia for Nurses and Nursing Students

Edited by Karen Harrison Dening. Foreword by Alistair Burns.

This essential textbook presents the wide range of issues faced by nurses and students working in dementia care. Grounded in high quality, up-to-date evidence, the book includes handy summaries and case studies to demonstrate the application of the evidence to practice.